KETO INTERMITTENT FASTING

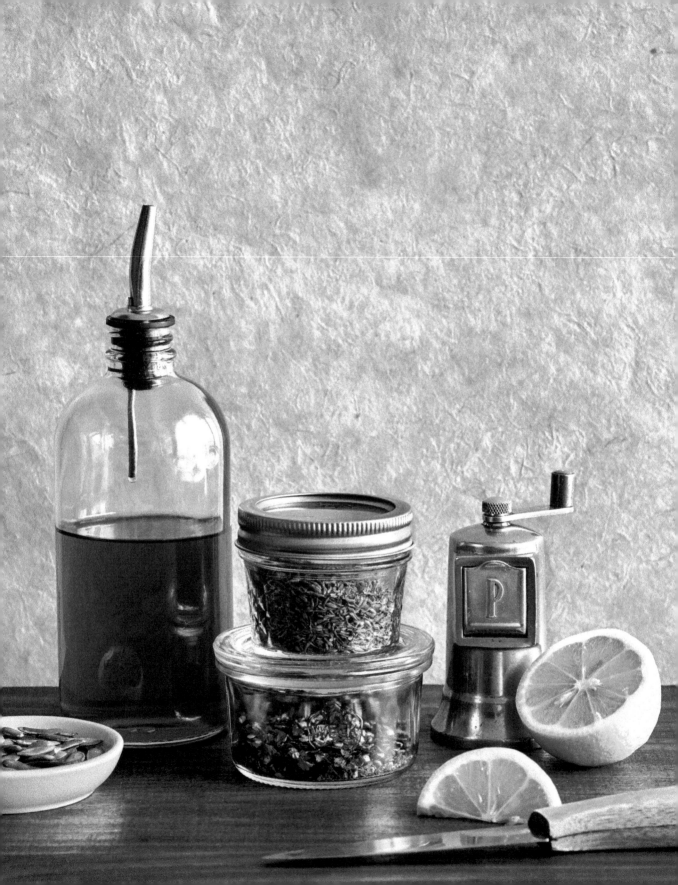

Keto Intermittent Fasting

100 High-Fat Low-Carb Recipes and Fasting Guidelines to Supercharge Your Health

BRIAN STANTON

WITH MICHELLE ANDERSON

PHOTOGRAPHY BY BIZ JONES

ROCKRIDGE
PRESS

For general information on our other products and services or to obtain technical support, please contact our Customer Care Department within the United States at (866) 744-2665, or outside the United States at (510) 253-0500.

Rockridge Press publishes its books in a variety of electronic and print formats. Some content that appears in print may not be available in electronic books, and vice versa.

TRADEMARKS: Rockridge Press and the Rockridge Press logo are trademarks or registered trademarks of Callisto Media Inc. and/or its affiliates, in the United States and other countries, and may not be used without written permission. All other trademarks are the property of their respective owners. Rockridge Press is not associated with any product or vendor mentioned in this book.

Interior and Cover Designer: Diana Haas
Art Producer: Michael Hardgrove
Editor: Laura Apperson
Production Editor: Ruth Sakata Corley
Photography © 2020 Biz Jones. Food styling by Erika Joyce..

ISBN: Print 978-1-64611-658-4 | eBook 978-1-64611-659-1
R0

For my mom and dad

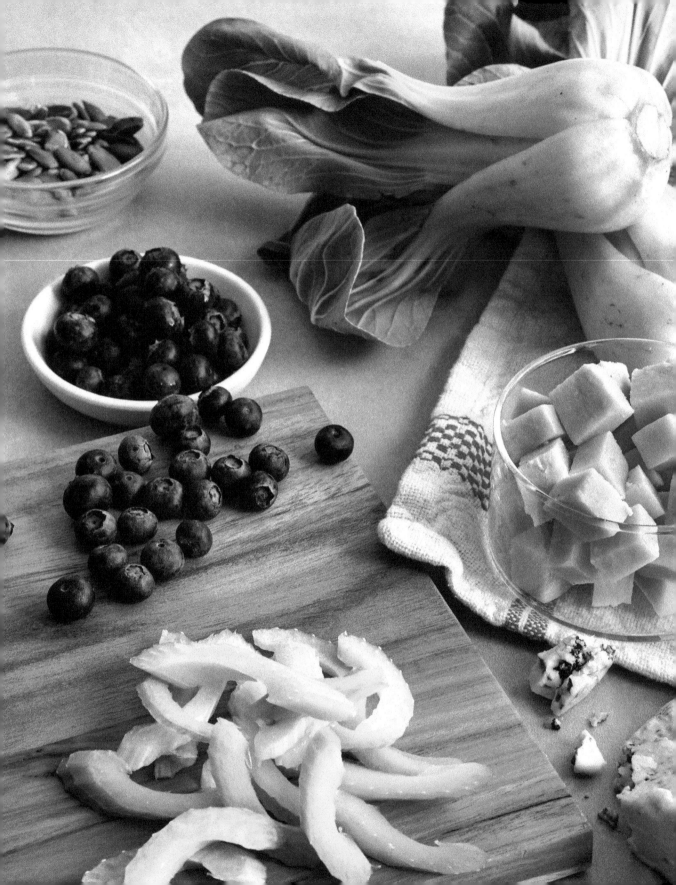

Contents

Introduction

YOU COULD BE DOING SOMETHING else right now. Instead of reading this book, you could be running errands, chatting with friends, or energetically googling your next getaway.

But you pressed pause on that stuff to crack open this keto fasting guide, and that says something special about you. It says you care about your health. Maybe your health is even your number one priority.

I hope that's the case. It will make getting results from this book much easier, not to mention gaining the benefit of living a longer, happier life.

I'm a big believer in putting health first, but my past self wasn't. I was the college student wolfing down double cheeseburgers and rubbery chicken sandwiches while most of the world slept. That was my weekend ritual. But when I turned 23, life intervened.

The intervention was a stomach virus. It lasted a week, but my symptoms lingered into May, June, July, and August. When I visited a gastroenterologist that summer, he nonchalantly diagnosed me with irritable bowel syndrome. The message was clear: I'd have these issues for life.

To say I was bummed would be an understatement. I was crushed. My thoughts spiraled into delusion, and I wished for my old body back. This unproductive mindset persisted for months as I zipped fruitlessly around the health-care system, visiting MDs, naturopaths, and even—I'm a bit sheepish to admit—a self-proclaimed "energy healer."

Finally, I took matters into my own hands. While I was supposed to be creating spreadsheets at work, I went deep on nutrition research. Keto wasn't popular yet, but a similar approach called Paleo was catching fire: no grains, no sugar, no processed junk—only foods we evolved to eat. I went all in.

I didn't get better overnight. It took time, effort, and experimentation, but over the course of many months, my symptoms faded to zero. Changing my diet cured me. It also propelled me into a highly rewarding career. I like to think that maybe my work is helping someone—someone like the 23-year-old me—who's ardently seeking better health.

You might be wondering how my story applies to keto and intermittent fasting.

It applies because diet is the single most important lever for managing your health. What you eat (and *when* you eat) has profound effects on your weight, energy levels, gut health, mood, and disease risk. Sleep, exercise, and social ties are close runners-up—and if you neglect these areas, your long-term health will suffer—but it all starts with diet.

The questions that need answering are simple: Why *this* diet? Why keto? Why intermittent fasting? The answer is also simple: They work.

I realize this is highly unpersuasive without supporting evidence. That's why I wrote chapter 1. There, you'll learn how keto fasting works to stimulate fat loss, increase focus, reduce cravings, and much more with lots of science and minimal jargon. Chapters 2 and 3 are more hands-on and are full of tools and meal plans (from recipe chapters 4 through 10) so that you can smoothly navigate various fasting protocols on the keto diet.

Keto fasting may seem restrictive, but you don't have to relinquish the joy of eating. By limiting your feeding time, you might even rekindle it.

Skeptical? That's understandable. The real persuasion will occur when you put the lessons of this book into practice and start seeing measurable improvements in your health.

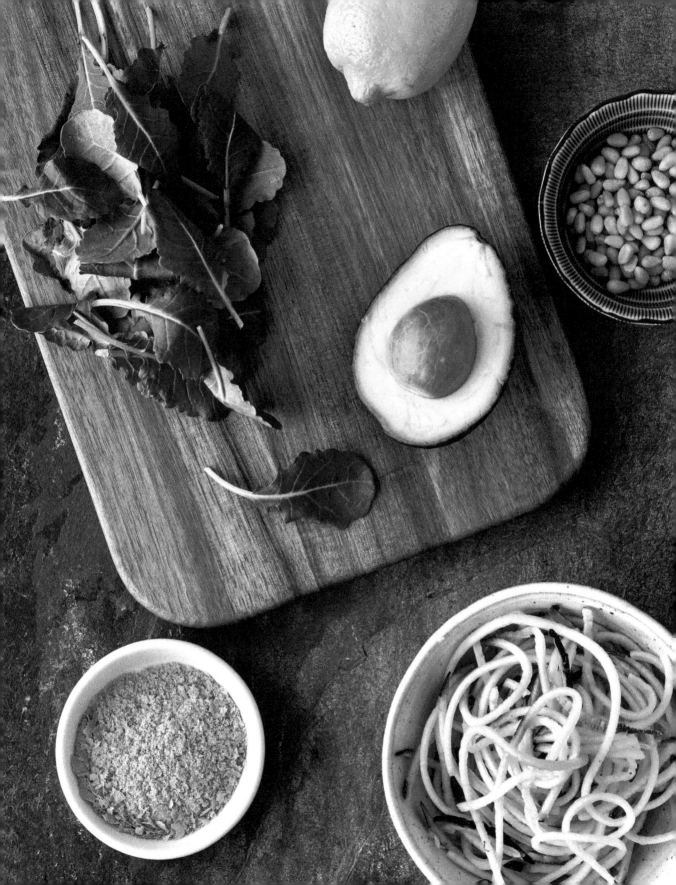

PART ONE

The Intermittent Fasting and Ketogenic Diet Lifestyle

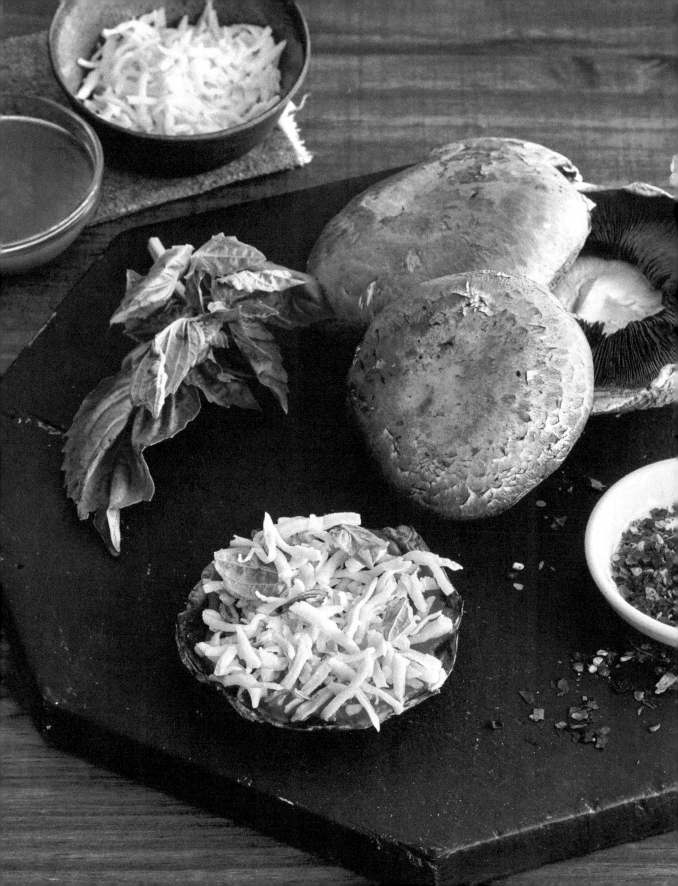

CHAPTER ONE

Your Intermittent Fasting and Keto Primer

Keto and intermittent fasting are not so different. On both regimens your body burns fat for energy.

Most diets don't have this effect. Most diets—especially high-carb diets—get you storing fat, not burning it. That's because most diets don't effectively lower insulin, your fat storage hormone. But when you fast, go keto, or both, your insulin levels drop. This is right where you want to be if you want to lose fat.

This book will help you combine intermittent fasting and keto, unleashing your inner fat burner. But before combining them, let's tackle them separately. Buckle in.

What Is Intermittent Fasting?

Intermittent fasting is a fancy term for a simple practice: taking regular breaks from eating food. That may not sound very scientific, but that's all intermittent fasting really is.

Some regimens are performed daily, others weekly. Some require calorie counting, while others don't. All these hairy details are covered in the next section.

This book focuses on intermittent fasting, not extended fasting. For our purposes, we'll call any fast more than 36 hours an *extended fast* and any fast between 12 and 36 hours an *intermittent fast*. If you've ever gone 12 hours between dinner and breakfast, congratulations: You've practiced intermittent fasting.

Fasting is nothing new. Twenty thousand years ago, our ancestors couldn't hit the store for fresh mammoth meat. They actually had to bring down a mammoth. When they failed at the hunt-and-gather game, they simply went without food.

Having evolved in such times, humans are marvelously adapted to periods of nutrient deprivation. That's because we have a rich energy source lining our anatomies: body fat, which is stored in molecules called triglycerides. During a fast, these triglycerides are split apart into fatty acids, which are subsequently burned for energy. That's what's happening when you lose fat on a fast.

This isn't just theoretical. According to a 2018 review in the medical science journal *Cureus*, multiple human studies have shown that intermittent fasting promotes significant fat loss.

Simply put, intermittent fasting unlocks a fat-burning system that has largely been silenced by our snack-happy culture. Fasting is convenient and simple to implement and works perfectly with the keto diet.

Types of Intermittent Fasting

First, let's be clear. Fasting is powerful medicine, but it's medicine without a directions label.

"Imagine you're some doctor . . . and someone hands you a bottle of pills and says, 'This is the single most valuable drug you have,'" remarked longevity expert Dr. Peter Attia. "And you're like, 'What's the dose?' 'I don't know.'"

It may take some trial and error to find the fasting dose that works best for you. This book will help guide you through that process.

To get you started, let's review the most popular forms of intermittent fasting. Keep these in mind when you select your fat-fueled meal plan in chapter 3.

DAILY FASTS

Daily fasting—or "time restricted feeding"—is the practice of eating all your food within a set time frame each day: no calorie restriction, just time restriction.

12/12

If you're new to intermittent fasting, 12/12 daily fasting is a good place to start.

The mechanics of 12/12 are simple. Just wait 12 hours between dinner and breakfast. For instance, stop eating at 7 p.m. and start eating again at 7 a.m.

An overnight fast is beneficial for two main reasons:

1. It keeps insulin low overnight because you aren't snacking.

2. It enhances your circadian rhythm, the 24-hour wake-sleep cycle that regulates your hormones, energy levels, mood, body weight . . . pretty much everything.

Eating at night sends wake-up signals to your body and should be avoided whenever possible. Fasting overnight helps you rest better and keeps your body humming along like the beautiful machine it is.

16/8

The next rung on the fasting ladder is called 16/8. When you practice 16/8, you eat all your calories within eight hours each day. The other 16 are fasting hours.

For instance, you might start the clock at 11 a.m. with a big breakfast and then shovel the last bite of dinner in your mouth at 7 p.m. Then you don't eat again until 11 a.m. the next day.

In a study published in the *Journal of Translational Medicine*, researchers found that eight weeks of 16/8 fasting reduced fat mass—but not muscle mass—in 34 athletic men.

One Meal a Day (OMAD)

Come Thanksgiving Day, I like to fast until the turkey is served. Then I'll eat about 4,000 calories (my normal caloric load), stagger to the living room, and watch football in a pleasantly full state.

That's One Meal a Day intermittent fasting, or OMAD. You eat *all* your calories in one sitting—at 8 a.m., 2 p.m., 6 p.m., or whenever you like, but preferably before the sun sets for circadian rhythm enhancement.

The key to getting results from OMAD is to stay near your normal daily calories. If you typically eat 2,000 calories a day, a 3,000-calorie feast won't move you closer to your health goals (unless you want to add weight).

A small study published in the *American Journal of Clinical Nutrition* found that OMAD led to significantly more fat loss than three-meal-a-day eating habits. And no, you don't need to restrict calories with OMAD.

WEEKLY FASTS

Weekly fasts alternate fasting and feeding days. Unlike daily fasting, weekly fasting involves calorie reduction on fasting days.

5:2

Of the weekly fasting protocols, 5:2 is the easiest to implement. You pick two nonconsecutive days each week (say, Monday and Thursday) to eat 20 percent to 25 percent of your normal caloric load. The other five days you eat per usual. This isn't the same as normal caloric restriction, which limits calories every day.

Here's how 5:2 works. If you usually eat 2,000 calories, you'll eat around 500 calories on fasting days. Fasting or not, try to eat all your calories in a 12-hour window, ideally while the sun is shining. I'll make this easy for you to implement in chapter 3.

Unsurprisingly, consuming significantly less food two days per week leads to significant weight loss. For example, a 2011 study published in the *International Journal of Obesity* found that overweight or obese women lost an average of 14.1 pounds after six months of 5:2 fasting.

Alternate-Day Modified Fasting (ADMF)

Similar to 5:2 is alternate-day modified fasting, or ADMF. Instead of limiting calories two days per week, you limit them every other day.

So, Monday you eat normally, Tuesday you eat 500 calories, Wednesday you are back to normal, and so on. There are many calorie restriction days, but on the bright side, you're always just a day away from a food party.

More importantly, ADMF works. A 2015 review across multiple studies found ADMF to be effective for promoting weight loss and improving markers of heart health.

Alternate-Day Fasting (ADF)

Alternate-day fasting (ADF) sits on the border between intermittent fasting and extended fasting. When you practice strict ADF, you eat *nothing* every other day. You go from Monday dinner to Wednesday breakfast—around 36 hours without food.

Alternate-day fasting is generally the hardest regimen for folks to comply with. It's tough being hungry every other day, not to mention the social difficulties.

But ADF is a powerful regimen. For example, fasting expert Dr. Jason Fung uses 36-hour ADF as part of his Intensive Dietary Management Program to treat type 2 diabetes.

Debunking Fasting Myths

For some, fasting evokes images of a shriveled castaway, devoid of muscle, marooned on a desert island for months without a proper meal. Yikes. But such a starved state would be due to caloric restriction, not intermittent fasting. So, before going any further, I'd like to debunk the three most common fasting myths.

MYTH #1: **Fasting is the same as caloric restriction.**
When you practice caloric restriction, you eat less food than your metabolism requires day after day, week after week. Yes, calorie restriction leads to weight loss, but it's also less sustainable and decreases the rate at which you use energy. The result is a cold, hungry human.

Intermittent fasting is more about restricting *when* you eat rather than *what* you eat. On feeding days and within feeding windows, you eat your fill.

MYTH #2: **Fasting makes you lose muscle.**
The research consistently shows that muscle is preserved during intermittent fasting. When your body needs energy during a fast, it reaches for fat stores, not lean mass. When that body fat gets burned, the resulting ketones also help preserve muscle.

Your body guards muscle like a mother penguin guards her chick. Think about it. Our ancestors wouldn't have lasted long if their strength evaporated during times of scarcity.

MYTH #3: **Fasting makes you overeat.**

At the end of a fast, you're going to be hungry. It's totally normal. Some worry, however, that this hunger will make you overeat in subsequent meals. Picture a starving hyena turned loose on a Chinese buffet.

But the science doesn't support this concern. In fact, most fasting studies permit ad libitum eating during feeding windows. In other words, folks eat as much as they like and *still* don't overdo the calories. Instead, they lose weight, drop fat, and see other metabolic improvements.

HOW MEN AND WOMEN FAST DIFFERENTLY

Both men and women have been fasting successfully since Paleolithic times. The human body, regardless of gender, will access stored body fat during a fast. Plenty of research supports this fact.

Some research, however, suggests small but noteworthy differences in how men and women respond to fasting. For instance, one study in *Behavioural Brain Research* documented a significant stress response in women after two days of fasting, while another study in *BioMed Research International* found the opposite response in men. (None of the regimens suggested in this book reach the 48-hour mark.)

In another study from the *Journal of Science and Medicine in Sport,* researchers from New Zealand found that male and female muscles adapted differently to exercise. Men did better in a fasted state, women in a fed state. Both men and women, though, showed improved VO2 max (that is, maximal oxygen uptake, a marker of endurance capacity) from the fasting protocol.

What about fasting and fertility? Well, extended fasting lowers fertility in both male and female rats—but in a study published in *Clinical Endocrinology*, a three-day fast didn't change the menstrual cycles of normal-weight women.

Finally, pregnant or nursing women should be cautious with fasts longer than 12 hours. There are too many important nutrients to pass along to the baby.

To be clear, intermittent fasting is safe and healthy for most people, including most women. But also keep in mind that fasting, like exercise, can be stressful. In the next chapter, we'll go into more detail on who shouldn't fast.

A good rule of thumb for both men and women is to start slowly and listen to your body. If you feel truly lousy (not just hungry), discontinue fasting and consider seeing a medical professional.

The Ketogenic Diet

The keto diet is a low-carb eating plan that—like intermittent fasting—gets you burning fat for energy. Keto is best known as a weight-loss diet, but having ketones in your blood has other benefits, too.

What Is Ketosis?

Ketosis is a unique metabolic state in which you rely less on sugar and more on fatty acids and ketones to supply your energy needs. These fatty acids (the precursor to ketones) come from either dietary fat or body fat, depending on how recently you've eaten. Fat, not sugar, powers your ketogenic state.

You have two main options for entering ketosis: fasting and the ketogenic diet. When you eat a keto diet, you ruthlessly restrict carbs to keep blood sugar low. Lower blood sugar leads to lower insulin levels, and low insulin is the key to ketosis.

"Hey, we're low on sugar!" says your body when insulin gets low. *"Time to start burning fat and making ketones."*

Ketones are tiny molecules, produced through beta-oxidizing (burning) fatty acids in the liver, that serve as a backup energy source to glucose. In particular, ketones help power your brain as you cruise through life in a low-sugar state.

If you're just starting a keto diet, how long will it take to start making ketones?

It depends. Some folks will enter ketosis overnight, while others may need a month or more to become a fat-burning machine. In general, the more your metabolism needs fixing, the longer it will take. Fasting accelerates the process. Nothing lowers insulin faster than eating nothing.

You can measure your level of ketosis through commercially available blood and urine tests, but don't get too hung up on these results. Rather, pay attention to whether you're losing fat, craving fewer carbs, and feeling unusually clearheaded—all positive signs you're in ketosis.

What Are Macros?

"Macros" is short for "macronutrients." The three macros—carbohydrates, protein, and fat—supply the raw materials for moving, breathing, growing, and healing.

Macronutrients come from two places: diet and body. You can eat fat, but you can also burn body fat for energy. Likewise, you can eat carbs, but you can also access stored carbs in your cells (called glycogen) to meet your glucose demands. And if your diet is consistently low in protein, you'll burn through your beautiful muscles to meet those needs.

On the ketogenic diet, macros matter. That's because keeping dietary carbs, fat, and protein in the right proportions keeps insulin low and sends the ketosis bat signal. Specifically, you want to eat 60 to 70 percent of your calories from fat, 20 to 30 percent from protein, and less than 10 percent from carbs. Let's take these one at a time.

Fat is your main macro on keto. Fat helps you build cell membranes, absorb fat soluble vitamins, and—yes—make ketones. Of all the macros, fat raises insulin the least, helping you stay in ketosis.

Next is protein. You need the building blocks of protein (amino acids) to form nearly every tissue in your body, including muscle. The research shows that moderate protein keto diets are perfectly compatible with weight loss, ketone production, and other keto-related benefits.

Finally, carbs. Restricting carbs is probably the hardest part of going keto, but it's nonnegotiable. Remember that low-carb means low blood sugar, low blood sugar means low insulin, and low insulin means fat-burning mode.

Put that last paragraph on your refrigerator. It's how ketosis happens.

But macros are only half the keto equation. The other half is food quality. For starters, your keto diet should be big on healthy fat and protein (such as olive oil, coconut oil, nuts, organic dairy, and pasture-raised meats) but small on peanut oil, soybean oil, and the rest of the inflammatory seed oil gang. Oh, and don't forget to eat your non-starchy vegetables. Your body will thank you.

The recipes in this book were designed with both macros and food quality in mind so that you don't have to worry about them.

CARB CYCLING

Carb cycling—also called keto cycling or cyclical keto—entails eating high-carb one or two days per week and strict keto all other days. Protein is held constant.

In terms of calories, high-carb days are around 10 percent fat, 25 percent protein, and 65 percent carbs. On low-carb days, your fat/protein/carb ratio returns to 65/25/10.

Should you carb cycle? That depends on your goals, activity level, and psychology.

Understand that eating high-carb *will* kick you out of ketosis. How quickly will you get back? That depends on how insulin sensitive you are. The more insulin sensitive you are, the less insulin you need to process the same amount of blood-sugar-raising carbohydrates. With less insulin around, you can reenter ketosis faster. For instance, an insulin-sensitive athlete might reenter ketosis hours after a carb refeed. A sedentary obese person, however, could take days to return to ketosis after eating carbs. That person needs more insulin to do the same job, and all that insulin prevents ketosis.

Most commonly, carb cycling is advertised as a performance enhancer for the serious low-carb athlete. The extra carbs, the theory goes, inject additional glucose into your system to fuel glycolytic (glucose-demanding) hard exercise.

But while carb cycling probably enhances some activities, such as marathons, it's by no means a requirement for most exercise. In fact, a study published in the *Journal of Strength and Conditioning Research* found that a strict keto diet improved strength, testosterone levels, and body composition in young men doing hard weight training.

The final benefit of carb cycling is psychological. Having a carb feast on the horizon can make keto more bearable. It's nice to have something to look forward to.

Go strict keto for at least a month before carb cycling. This will accelerate your fat adaptation (your body's ability to burn fat for energy), allowing you to return to ketosis faster after carb refeeds.

Intermittent Fasting and Keto: A Power Couple

Intermittent fasting and keto are more or less the same diet. During a fast, you burn body fat, and after eating a keto-friendly meal, you burn dietary fat.

In both cases, your cells get used to burning fat. Because of this, combining keto and fasting creates a diet more powerful than either alone. Ah, synergy.

Introducing Your New Fat-Burning State

Imagine your body has a toggle switch that indicates how you're using energy. One side says "store," and the other says "burn." Are you storing calories for later, or are you burning them now?

Lording over this switch is insulin—the boss energy hormone. The more insulin that's around, the more the dial shifts to storage mode. All foods increase insulin, but carbs have the greatest effect. Protein spikes insulin less than carbs do, and fat even less.

Let's say you eat a high-carb meal. Blood sugar rises, and insulin surges to remove the excess glucose from your bloodstream. First, insulin attempts to store it as glycogen, but only about 500 grams of carbs can be stored in liver and muscle tissue. This is your glycogen tank, and it fills up quickly. It's like the overhead compartment on an airplane. But insulin isn't worried about running out of space; there's plenty of room below the main cabin. When the overhead bin gets full, insulin doesn't hesitate to check your bag as body fat.

Basically, high insulin equals fat-storage mode. For many folks, insulin stays high week after week, month after month, leading to a permanent fat-storage mode.

Here's why: When you eat frequently (especially carbs), insulin keeps surging, and your cells eventually stop listening to insulin. This condition, called insulin resistance, means insulin stays high, blood sugar stays high, weight stays high, and chronic disease risk increases. Insulin resistance, in fact, is the defining feature of type 2 diabetes.

Let's go back to the toggle switch. To move the dial to "burn," you need to keep insulin low. When it comes to lowering insulin and breaking the cycle of insulin resistance, you have two main dietary options: fasting and keto.

In study after study, both keto dieting and intermittent fasting have been shown to lower insulin. With insulin low, your cells can finally access the cargo sequestered deep in the belly of the plane: body fat.

It's easy to understand how fasting gets you burning fat. No food means no insulin response. Then you start using fat instead of glucose for energy.

The keto diet is similar to fasting, but with dietary fat. Dietary fat raises insulin very little, helping you avoid fat storage mode. This is why keto is so effective for reversing type 2 diabetes.

Together, keto and intermittent fasting are a power couple. Both diets get you running on fat and making ketones. When combined, they shove you into fat-burning mode faster than either alone.

If you're struggling to get results from keto, adding intermittent fasting to the mix could make a meaningful difference. Likewise, if fasting seems unbearable right now, pairing it with a keto diet could accelerate your fat loss and mitigate your hunger. In fact, a study published in the *European Journal of Clinical Nutrition* found that a ketogenic diet helped suppress ghrelin (the hunger hormone) in 50 people during a weight-loss protocol.

When combining intermittent fasting and keto, here are some rules to keep in mind:

- Eat within a set time frame each day (12 hours maximum).

- Don't limit calories, unless the fasting protocol calls for it.

- Eat high-fat, moderate-protein, and low-carb meals (65/25/10 ratio).

- Minimize snacking to minimize insulin.

   If you need extra motivation to get started, keep reading.

Two Is Better Than One: Health Benefits

You just learned why fasting and the keto diet are a power couple. They work together to get you burning—not storing—fat. This can lead to healthy weight loss, of course, but research shows there are other health benefits, too.

WEIGHT LOSS

As standalone regimens, both keto and intermittent fasting have helped many people lose weight. For instance, one study in the *American Journal of Clinical Nutrition* found that modified alternate-day fasting helped non-obese people lose 11 more pounds than controls over 12 weeks. And in a 2003 controlled study, a six-month keto diet was shown to promote more weight loss than a calorie-restricted diet in obese women.

Absorb that for a moment. The women practicing keto ate *more* calories and still lost more weight. That's because calorie counting isn't the key to weight loss—keeping blood sugar and insulin low is.

REVERSING INSULIN RESISTANCE

When you're insulin resistant, you can't effectively store blood sugar. As a result, your blood sugar and insulin levels stay high, which in turn promotes fat storage. Every chronic disease is associated with this state: heart disease, cancer, Alzheimer's disease, you name it.

This is where keto and fasting come in. Both not only lower insulin levels but also improve insulin function. They're powerful medicines for reversing type 2 diabetes.

There's still widespread confusion about the dietary management of insulin resistance, but the tide may be turning. In fact, a recent consensus report in the journal *Diabetes Care* recommended carbohydrate reduction as the dietary intervention with the "most evidence" for helping diabetics manage blood sugar levels.

STABLE ENERGY

Fat-burning mode isn't just about shedding excess pounds. It's also about changing the way you power your day.

When you fat-adapt instead of riding the blood sugar roller coaster, you ride the smooth and steady fat train. On the fat train, you can cruise comfortably for hours without food. Breakfast can be skipped (maybe even lunch), and there's no more four o'clock slump.

Adapting to fat for energy won't happen overnight, but combining keto and intermittent fasting will accelerate the process.

REDUCED CRAVINGS

You'll get hungry when you fast. This is healthy and normal. But to be clear, your hunger shouldn't get out of control because running on fat puts the brakes on your hunger hormone, ghrelin. And when you *do* eat, you'll feel fuller for longer because fat and protein fill you up better than carbs.

BRAIN HEALTH

When you fast or go keto, you produce ketones. Ketones, in turn, fuel the brain when glucose is scarce. In a study published in the journal *Psychopharmacology*, researchers found that elevating blood ketone levels with medium chain triglyceride (MCT) oil led to improved cognitive function in elderly adults. Other researchers speculate that ketosis may be therapeutic for people with Alzheimer's disease, though human trials are lacking.

GUT HEALTH

Your gut likes to take breaks from food. Fasting allows the gut barrier to heal and regenerate. In fact, a study published in the journal *Cell Stem Cell* found that extended fasting regenerated intestinal cells in mice. Depending on your situation, keto can improve gut health, too. In his 2018 book *Healthy Gut, Healthy You*, Dr. Michael Ruscio recommended a low-carb diet for treating small intestinal bacterial overgrowth (SIBO), a condition underlying many chronic gut diseases. Removing carbs starves the bad bacteria, allowing your gut microbiome to rebalance itself.

LONGEVITY

Fasting activates a process called *autophagy* in your cells. During autophagy, your cells clean themselves, digesting old parts and replacing them with new ones. Think of it as an antiaging cellular restoration program. Longer fasts induce more autophagy than shorter ones, but because most of the evidence is in animals, we still don't know the best protocol for humans.

A keto diet may also activate autophagy. The evidence is preliminary, but in rats, a ketogenic diet induced autophagy and protected their brains from seizure-induced injury.

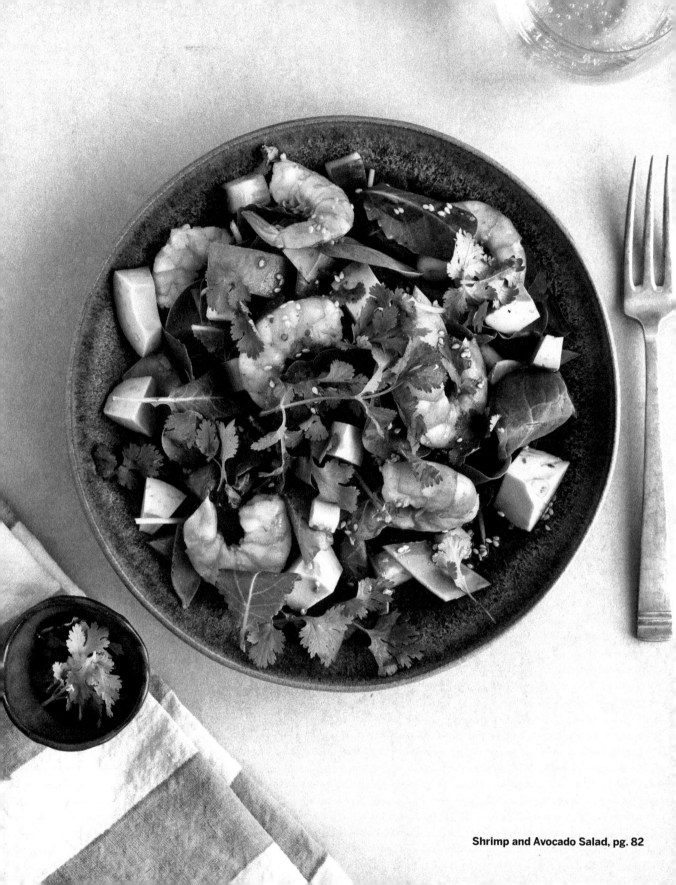

Shrimp and Avocado Salad, pg. 82

CHAPTER TWO

How to Prepare for Your Fast with Keto

If you've never fasted before, going more than 12 hours without food can be a struggle. To ease this transition, start your keto diet first. Going keto helps you fat-adapt, allowing you to access body fat during your fasts.

Before You Begin

Before we cover specific keto meal planning, there's some practical knowledge to cover on both fasting and keto.

Who Can and Cannot Fast?

Fasting is safe for most people, but there are exceptions. The following groups should not, under any circumstances, fast.

ANYONE WHO IS UNDERWEIGHT. When people are underweight (a body mass index under 18.5), they're at increased risk for heart disease, muscle loss, and bone density issues. Underweight folks need to gain weight, not lose weight, so fasting is a bad idea.

ANYONE STRUGGLING WITH AN EATING DISORDER. Those with a history of anorexia or bulimia need to mend their relationship with food and increase caloric intake. Fasting won't help accomplish these goals.

PREGNANT AND NURSING WOMEN. There's a reason a woman gets ravenous when pregnant: She's eating for two. This hunger is a signal to provide much-needed nutrients to the growing fetus. When the baby is born, nutrient requirements remain high to support breastfeeding. If a woman is deficient in nutrients such as folate, vitamin D, vitamin B$_{12}$, calcium, or magnesium, the quality of her breast milk will suffer. Fasting is not recommended.

GROWING CHILDREN. Fasting isn't a growth-promoting strategy. That's because fasting may, intentionally or not, lead to calorie or nutrient deficiencies. (Protein, iron, calcium, zinc, and folate are especially important to fuel growth spurts.) This doesn't mean children should be encouraged to snack constantly. Snacking at night, for instance, will disrupt their circadian clocks. Just provide healthy, satiating foods at normal mealtimes, and be stingy with the Froot Loops.

And these folks should have a chat with their doctors before fasting:

PEOPLE TAKING CERTAIN MEDICATIONS. According to Dr. Jason Fung, aspirin, metformin, iron, and magnesium supplements may cause issues during a fast. These medications are best taken with food to avoid gastrointestinal distress. Also, metformin and injectable insulin decrease blood sugar levels and raise the risk of hypoglycemia (dangerously low blood sugar) during a fast. If you're taking any medications, consult your doctor before fasting.

DIABETICS. Properly managed, fasting can ameliorate both type 1 and 2 diabetes. Without supervision, however, diabetics run the risk of developing hypoglycemia, which can be fatal if blood sugar levels aren't quickly restored. Talk to your doctor about structuring a fasting program if you have type 1 diabetes, type 2 diabetes, or any other chronic condition.

Understand that fasting, like exercise, is a stressor. If you're already stressed from illness, sleep deprivation, work, or personal problems, think long and hard before adding any fast longer than 12 hours to that list. Picture your stress capacity as a water bottle. How full is your stress bottle? Is there room for fasting in there? If there's room, go for it. But if not, don't sweat it. Just work on your sleep, work stress, etc., and return to fasting another time.

I have a simple rule: If I don't sleep well the night before, I don't fast. My body is already stressed enough. There's no need to stress it further.

When you *do* fast, pay special attention to how you feel. Hunger is normal, but feeling shaky or faint is not. When in doubt, break the fast.

COMMON SIDE EFFECTS OF INTERMITTENT FASTING AND KETO

Along your keto fasting path, you may hit some snags. Here are the most common:

HUNGER: Hunger during fasting isn't as scary as you might imagine. We'll cover hunger and how to deal with it in the next section.

KETO FLU: When you remove carbs from your diet, your body may protest. This protest—which takes the form of headaches, fatigue, and mood swings—is commonly called the "keto flu." Keto flu is often a case of sugar withdrawal. Similar to caffeine, your body gets addicted to sugar, and going cold turkey can be painful. This should pass as you enter ketosis. Be aware, however, that electrolyte deficiencies (especially low sodium) and dehydration can also cause keto flu symptoms.

KETO BREATH: Keto dieters often report fruity-smelling breath. This strange side effect is likely due to acetone—a type of ketone—present in saliva. Fortunately, keto breath is easily remedied with mints, gum, or peppermint oil.

GUT PROBLEMS: Both fasting and keto limit dietary fiber, which may affect bowel habits. Assuming they don't cause gut distress, eat plenty of non-starchy vegetables to increase fiber intake and stay regular. Digestive issues may also result from shifts in gut bacteria, dehydration, or sensitivities to new foods in your diet.

SLEEP ISSUES: Early on, eliminating carbs may cause insomnia, a classic carb-withdrawal symptom. Also, fasting increases adrenaline, which can make it harder to wind down. If you're struggling to sleep at night, consider exercising more during the day, getting lots of light in the morning, and limiting blue light at night. If all else fails, you can also retreat to an easier fasting regimen.

MUSCLE CRAMPS: If you're cramping during keto or fasting, look first to electrolytes. In particular, you may need more salt because (1) your fat-burning, low-insulin state signals your kidneys to excrete extra sodium and (2) whole foods are naturally low in salt. In other words, your sodium intake is low, and your sodium excretion is high. Increase salt intake by salting your food or by taking an electrolyte supplement that contains sodium.

As always, if you're concerned about these side effects, chat with your doctor before fasting.

Overcoming Hunger

Hunger is the bogeyman of intermittent fasting. It is widely feared but rarely dangerous. Many folks worry that during a fast, hunger will continue spiraling upward, ad infinitum. *If I'm this hungry after 12 hours, how will I feel after 16?*

The truth is you'll probably feel about the same. In one study, a 36-hour fast and a 12-hour fast affected ghrelin—the hunger hormone—roughly equally. In other words, hunger stabilizes over time.

Let's double-click on ghrelin for a moment. Ghrelin is secreted in your stomach, stimulates cravings, and makes you want that snack oh so badly. Many things affect ghrelin and therefore hunger. Take sleep, for instance: One controlled study showed that two nights of short sleep (four hours) significantly increased both ghrelin and appetite in humans. The keto diet, on the other hand, has been shown to reduce circulating ghrelin levels. More fat means less hunger hormone.

Keto, however, is more than just a ghrelin reducer. Low-carb diets also:

- decrease an appetite-stimulating brain factor called neuropeptide Y and

- increase a satiety hormone called cholecystokinin (CCK).

This hunger-management benefit of keto carries over into fasting periods. It's a big reason why these diets work so well together.

Yet keto or not, you'll still get hungry during a fast. It's like driving home during rush hour. No matter what route you take, you're going to hit traffic.

Much of hunger, in fact, is driven by habit and conditioning. Let me share a personal example.

These days, I don't usually get hungry until 10 or 11 a.m. That's because I eat around that time every day. It's become a habit, and my hunger response is now synced with my routine.

Certain cues, however, can activate my hunger response earlier. Sometimes I'll catch a whiff of grilled meat from the burger joint down the road. When that happens, the time of day doesn't matter. Saliva fills my mouth, my stomach starts rumbling, and I become a ravenous beast.

Something similar happens to everyone. Maybe you see your favorite dessert in the freezer, then all of a sudden—WHAM—a conditioned hunger response sets in. The conditioned response doesn't care that you just ate dinner. You crave that ice cream anyway.

Overcoming hunger, then, requires a bit of planning. Here are some tips.

MIND YOUR ENVIRONMENT. Remove obvious hunger cues (such as visible food) to avoid conditioned hunger responses.

RIDE IT OUT. Hunger ebbs and flows during a fast. If you're super hungry, hang in there. It should pass within an hour or less.

KEEP OCCUPIED. Schedule your day to avoid downtime. A focused mind hasn't time to bother with hunger.

SLEEP WELL. Short sleep increases ghrelin, your hunger hormone.

EAT KETO DURING FEEDING WINDOWS. Keto dieting curbs hunger and helps you access body fat during a fast.

SUBSTITUTE LOW-CALORIE OPTIONS. Drinking tea, coffee, or broth can help maintain ritual and soothe your brain as you count down the seconds to mealtime. The handful of calories from broth shouldn't meaningfully affect the benefits of your fast. Flip to chapter 9 for low-calorie drink recipes.

11 Tips for Success with Intermittent Fasting and Keto

With your hunger strategy firmly in place, here are 11 practical tips to help you navigate your keto-fueled fasting journey.

1. **GO KETO FIRST.** Becoming a fat burner doesn't happen overnight. Your body needs time to fat-adapt. To facilitate this adaptation, try a week or two of keto dieting as an initial step. This will get you running on fat for fuel and make your transition to intermittent fasting much smoother.

2. **FIND YOUR FASTING PROTOCOL.** If you're a novice faster, start with 12/12 (see page 5) and work your way up. Perhaps a 12-hour fast is your sweet spot, but feel free to experiment. Personally, I like 16/8.

As a general rule, longer fasts will stimulate more rapid weight loss, but there's no need to be a hero. If you can't tolerate anything longer than a 14-hour fast, don't sweat it. You'll still get benefits with shorter fasts. In the next chapter, you'll learn the baby-step method of intermittent fasting. This will help you choose the right fasting protocol while minimizing discomfort along the way.

3. **EAT YOUR FILL, BUT DON'T GORGE YOURSELF.** Weekly fasting protocols such as 5:2 (see page 6) limit calories on fasting days. During feeding windows, however, you should eat your fill to prevent nutrient deficiencies. "Eat your fill" is the operative term here. Before jumping up for seconds or thirds, give your body 20 to 30 minutes to feel full after a meal. This allows time for your satiety hormone, leptin, to kick in. If you stuff yourself beyond capacity, your gut will pay the price, and you'll wish you had eaten less. Overeating can also hinder weight-loss goals.

4. **TRACK METRICS.** As the old business maxim goes, "What gets measured, gets managed." How can you measure your progress? For starters, use urine or blood ketone test strips to confirm you're in ketosis. More importantly, monitor functional metrics such as weight loss, personal energy, and focus. These should always be improving, at least on a weekly basis. If they're not, refer back to these tips for success.

5. **EAT NON-STARCHY VEGETABLES.** Keto and intermittent fasting are both restrictive. On the keto fasting program, you have fewer hours to eat fewer types of food. To prevent vitamin and mineral deficiencies, look to non-starchy vegetables to fill the empty space on your plate. (Specific food recommendations will come later in this chapter.)

6. **EAT HEALTHY FATS.** Vegetables alone won't cut it. Your keto plate should also be full of healthy fats such as olive oil, coconut oil, and animal fat. These fats are not only nutritious but also keep insulin low so that you can stay in fat-burning mode. Avoid unhealthy fats such as peanut oil, soybean oil, and other high-omega-6 vegetable oils like your life depends on it.

7. **TAKE ELECTROLYTES.** Electrolytes such as sodium, potassium, magnesium, and calcium allow nerve impulses to fire, muscles to function, and blood to flow. Low-carb folks need more electrolytes because:

- low-carb diets restrict many electrolyte-rich foods (e.g., fruit and potatoes) and

- you pee out more sodium in a low-insulin state.

Bottom line? Salt your food aggressively and consider supplementing with magnesium and potassium.

8. **STAY HYDRATED.** Along with sodium, your kidneys excrete more water in a low-insulin state. To keep hydrated, drink a glass of water when you wake up, and drink to thirst throughout the day. Don't expect water to fill you up, though. Your body is smarter than that.

9. **DRINK COFFEE, TEA, OR BROTH.** These beverages tend to cut hunger better than water. Compounds in coffee and tea can curb your appetite, and broth has satiating calories from collagen protein. See chapters 9 and 5, respectively, for recipes.

10. **PLAN AHEAD.** Don't rely on willpower to muscle through your keto fasting program. Write everything down, including mealtimes and meal composition, and stick to your schedule. When something's on a piece of paper, you're more likely to follow through. You'll also find that constraining your choices with a set schedule makes life easier. Fewer decisions means less decision fatigue.

11. **REMOVE TEMPTATIONS.** Go through your kitchen and throw out any carby, sugary, or otherwise unhealthy food that might tempt you or trigger a conditioned hunger response. If this isn't possible, hide them somewhere. Out of sight, out of mind.

The Keto Kitchen

It's time to prep your kitchen for keto. In this section, I include foods to buy and foods to chuck, instructions on how to structure your plate, and the ingredients you'll need to keep in the kitchen. I even provide a few words on equipment.

This will take effort at first, but once you're all set up, maintenance will be minimal.

Knowing What to Eat

Going keto means eating high-fat, moderate-protein, low-carb meals. It also means avoiding anything processed. Read on for specific food recommendations.

FOODS TO LOVE

Keto isn't as restrictive as you might think. Yes, you need to eliminate most carbs, but there's a long list of delicious, nutritious foods to take their place. Focus on the following categories when structuring your plates.

Fats and Oils

Superstar: extra-virgin olive oil. Olive oil is high in monounsaturated fat, contains the powerful antioxidant oleuropein, and has been shown in numerous studies to improve heart disease risk markers.

- ❑ Avocado oil
- ❑ Butter
- ❑ Coconut butter
- ❑ Egg yolks
- ❑ Extra-virgin olive oil
- ❑ Ghee
- ❑ Lard
- ❑ Macadamia nut oil
- ❑ MCT oil
- ❑ Organic unrefined red palm oil
- ❑ Sesame oil
- ❑ Tallow
- ❑ Walnut oil

Nuts and Seeds

Superstar: macadamia nut. Of all the nuts, macadamia has the lowest omega-6-to-omega 3-ratio. Researchers believe that lowering this ratio can help lower inflammation and obesity risk.

- ❑ Almonds
- ❑ Brazil nuts
- ❑ Cashews
- ❑ Coconut meat (shredded or whole)
- ❑ Hazelnuts
- ❑ Macadamia nut
- ❑ Nut butter (with any of these nuts)
- ❑ Pecans
- ❑ Pistachios
- ❑ Pumpkin seeds
- ❑ Sunflower seeds
- ❑ Tahini (sesame seed paste)
- ❑ Walnuts

Proteins

Superstar: egg. The egg is the ideal keto food: high fat, medium protein, and very low-carb. Plus egg yolks are rich in important nutrients such as choline and vitamin A.

- ❑ Beef
- ❑ Collagen protein powder
- ❑ Egg
- ❑ Fish (includes cod, salmon, tuna, mackerel, cod, mahi mahi, and red snapper)
- ❑ Lamb
- ❑ Organ meats (includes liver, kidney, and heart)
- ❑ Pork
- ❑ Poultry (includes chicken, duck, and turkey)
- ❑ Shellfish (includes shrimp, clams, oysters, and lobster)
- ❑ Vegan protein options (includes pea protein, hemp protein, tofu, vegan cheese, and tempeh)
- ❑ Whey protein powder

Dairy Products

Note: Many folks don't react well to lactose (milk sugar) or casein (milk protein) in these foods. If you're one of these people, feel free to use almond and coconut products in recipes calling for dairy.

Superstar: butter. Butter is high in vitamins A, D, and K as well as the anti-inflammatory compound butyrate. Get your butter from pasture-raised cows for maximum nutrition.

- ❑ Butter
- ❑ Cheese (includes cream cheese, goat cheese, feta, gouda, mozzarella, and Brie)
- ❑ Heavy cream
- ❑ Whole raw milk
- ❑ Yogurt

Non-Starchy Vegetables

Note: This list isn't comprehensive because there are too many vegetables to name. As a general rule, look for vegetables with under 5 grams of net carbs per serving (you want to stay under about 20 grams of net carbs per day).

Superstar: kale. Kale is rich in vitamin K, the antioxidants lutein and zeaxanthin, and isothiocyanates—compounds with promising anticancer effects.

- ❑ Arugula
- ❑ Asparagus
- ❑ Bok choy
- ❑ Broccoli
- ❑ Brussels sprouts
- ❑ Cabbage
- ❑ Cauliflower
- ❑ Kale
- ❑ Mushrooms
- ❑ Romaine lettuce
- ❑ Spinach
- ❑ Watercress

Flavorings and Sweeteners

Superstar: erythritol. Noncaloric and a potent antioxidant, erythritol doesn't raise blood sugar and insulin levels like most other sweeteners.

- ❏ Cocoa powder
- ❏ Erythritol
- ❏ Monk fruit
- ❏ Stevia
- ❏ Vanilla extract

Beverages

Superstar: green tea. Compounds in green tea called catechins may help stimulate weight loss by increasing metabolic rate.

- ❏ Almond milk
- ❏ Black tea
- ❏ Broth
- ❏ Coffee
- ❏ Green tea
- ❏ Hemp milk
- ❏ Herbal tea
- ❏ Lemon juice
- ❏ Sparkling water

FOODS TO EAT IN MODERATION

Foods to limit on keto include the following.

- ❏ Alcohol: Alcohol won't help your keto goals, but the occasional serving of wine or hard alcohol (both low-carb) should be fine. Strive to avoid concoctions with added sugar, though.
- ❏ Avocados: This fruit is high in fiber, monounsaturated fat, and vitamin E, but it also contains 12 grams of carbs. Limit to one per day.
- ❏ Berries (includes blueberries, raspberries, cranberries, and blackberries): These fruits are low in sugar and high in antioxidants. You can have a few berries, but keep portions small to limit carbs.
- ❏ Dark chocolate: Shoot for at least 85 percent cacao bars with minimal added sugar.
- ❏ Tomatoes: Though high in the antioxidant lutein, tomatoes also have about 5 grams of carbs per fruit.

FOODS TO ELIMINATE

Get the donation bag ready. Here are foods that don't belong in your keto kitchen.

Grains

Why avoid? Grains contain too many carbs for keto. Grains also contain compounds such as gluten, phytic acid, and lectins that damage the gut and block nutrient absorption.

- ❏ Barley
- ❏ Bread
- ❏ Corn
- ❏ Millet
- ❏ Oats
- ❏ Pasta
- ❏ Quinoa
- ❏ Rice
- ❏ Rye

Starchy Vegetables

Why avoid? These foods aren't unhealthy per se, but they'll spike insulin and keep you from entering ketosis.

- ❏ Beets
- ❏ Carrots
- ❏ Parsnips
- ❏ Potatoes
- ❏ Sweet potatoes
- ❏ Turnips

Sugary Fruits

Why avoid? Except for berries, avocados, lemons, and limes, most fruits are too high in fructose (sugar) to make the keto cut.

- ❏ Apples
- ❏ Bananas
- ❏ Cherries
- ❏ Grapes
- ❏ Kiwifruit
- ❏ Melon (all types)
- ❏ Oranges
- ❏ Peaches
- ❏ Plums

Anything with Added Sugar

Why avoid? Sugar raises insulin levels and prevents fat-burning. In other words, sugar is the nemesis of ketosis.

Pro tip: To avoid refined sugar, shop the periphery of the grocery store. If it comes in a package, there's probably sugar in it.

- ❏ Candy
- ❏ Cookies
- ❏ Crackers
- ❏ Granola bars
- ❏ Juice
- ❏ Salad dressing
- ❏ Soda
- ❏ Tomato sauce

Industrial Seed Oils

Why avoid? These vegetable oils are high in the inflammatory omega-6 fat linoleic acid. Researchers believe that excessive linoleic acid consumption is partly responsible for the American obesity epidemic.

Pro tip: Avoid cooking with these unstable oils. They oxidize when heated, forming compounds called oxidized lipids, which drive the progression of heart disease.

- ❑ Canola oil
- ❑ Corn oil
- ❑ Cottonseed oil
- ❑ Peanut oil
- ❑ Safflower oil
- ❑ Soybean oil
- ❑ Sunflower oil

Processed Meats

Why avoid? These highly processed foods contain added sugar, artificial ingredients, and preservatives. They give meat a bad name.

- ❑ Ham
- ❑ Hot dogs
- ❑ Lunch meats
- ❑ Pepperoni

Artificial Sweeteners

Why avoid? A study published in the journal *Diabetes Care* found that drinking just one artificially sweetened soda per day is associated with a 67 percent higher risk of type 2 diabetes.

- ❑ Acesulfame potassium
- ❑ Aspartame
- ❑ Saccharine
- ❑ Sucralose

Planning Your Macros

Keto meal planning may seem daunting, but it's easier than you think. In fact, every recipe in this book was formulated to be keto-friendly. Just plug and play.

If you want to deviate from the recipes, that's easy, too. You just need to mind your macros.

Recall from chapter 1 that your keto diet should be around 65 percent fat, 25 percent protein, and 10 percent carbs. Keeping carbs low and fat high shoves you into ketosis, while eating moderate amounts of protein helps you maintain muscle mass.

You should be structuring your meals to be high in fat, moderate in protein, and full of non-starchy vegetables. Add a few berries and an avocado to the mix, and you'll be hitting your macro targets nicely.

When in doubt, combine eggs with leafy greens for a quick and easy keto calorie bomb. You can also use leafy greens as a base for protein and fat calories. Most people call this a salad.

In general, be liberal with your healthy fats. Dump them on everything. From time to time, I've even been known to drink olive oil directly from the bottle. Not only is this a big time-saver, but a spoonful of healthy fat can also provide energy during a fast without kicking you out of ketosis.

In the beginning, tracking macros with an app such as Chronometer can be useful, but don't stress about hitting exact percentages. Once you learn the caloric breakdown of your favorite keto foods, you can ballpark your plates. Finally, use ketone test strips occasionally to confirm you're on track, and then make adjustments as needed.

Curating Your Kitchen

This section covers what you need to make your keto recipes. Get the shopping list ready.

PANTRY ESSENTIALS

It's time to stock your pantry with keto-friendly fare. When buying the listed items, shoot for organic and unprocessed options whenever possible. This will minimize your toxic load while maximizing your nutrition.

HERBS AND SPICES

❑ Black pepper

❑ Chili powder

❑ Cinnamon, ground

❑ Cumin, ground

❑ Oregano, dried

❑ Salt (Himalayan pink salt is a good option)

❑ Thyme, dried

NUT FLOUR

❑ Almond flour

- ❏ Apple cider vinegar
- ❏ Balsamic vinegar
- ❏ Extra-virgin olive oil
- ❏ Sesame oil
- ❏ Virgin unrefined coconut oil

SWEETENERS AND FLAVORINGS

- ❏ Cocoa powder
- ❏ Granulated erythritol
- ❏ Vanilla extract

REFRIGERATED ESSENTIALS

Keep these refrigerated items handy for whipping up keto meals and snacks at a moment's notice.

- ❏ Almond milk: high-fat, dairy-free base for smoothies
- ❏ Broth: use chicken, beef, or fish stock (see chapter 5 for broth recipes)
- ❏ Butter: rich in vitamin A and low in lactose and casein
- ❏ Cheese: feta, Cheddar, Swiss, goat, blue—whatever you like
- ❏ Chicken: ultra-versatile protein source
- ❏ Coconut milk: rich in lauric acid and beneficial medium chain tri-glycerides (MCTs)
- ❏ Eggs: nutrient dense, eggs are absolute keto essentials
- ❏ Heavy cream: for keto soups, pastas, and desserts (coconut cream can be substituted)
- ❏ Kale: an antioxidant-rich superfood
- ❏ Spinach: for folate, potassium, and beta-carotene

OTHER PERISHABLE ESSENTIALS

And here's a short list of other fruits, nuts, and snacks to stock your kitchen with.

- ❏ Almonds
- ❏ Avocados
- ❏ Basil, fresh
- ❏ Garlic, fresh
- ❏ Hemp hearts
- ❏ Lemons
- ❏ Limes
- ❏ Parsley, fresh
- ❏ Pecans
- ❏ Tomatoes

NOTES ON SWEETENERS

Sweetening is allowed on keto. Just be sure to sweeten wisely.

Shirk sugar, of course, but also avoid artificial sweeteners such as aspartame, saccharine, or sucralose. They all provoke an insulin response that will hamper fat-burning goals.

Favor natural zero-calorie sweeteners such as stevia, monk fruit, and erythritol, which have minimal impact on blood sugar and insulin levels.

EQUIPMENT

If you cook frequently, you probably already have the cookware to become a certified keto chef. But if not, you may need to pick up a few items.

When selecting your cookware, pay close attention to the materials used. You'll want to avoid anything with nonstick coating such as Teflon. This coating leaches into food (and surrounding air) when heated, posing a potential health hazard.

Also, try to minimize plastic usage, especially when storing hot food. This will lower your exposure to BPA, among other dangerous chemicals. Start converting your kitchen to stainless-steel, cast iron, and glass cookware instead. It may cost a few extra dollars, but your health is worth it.

Armed with the following equipment, you can knock out most of the recipes in this book.

- ❏ Baking dish
- ❏ Baking sheet
- ❏ Blender
- ❏ Food storage containers
- ❏ Large skillet or wok
- ❏ Large stockpot
- ❏ Medium saucepan
- ❏ Mixing bowls

Happy cooking.

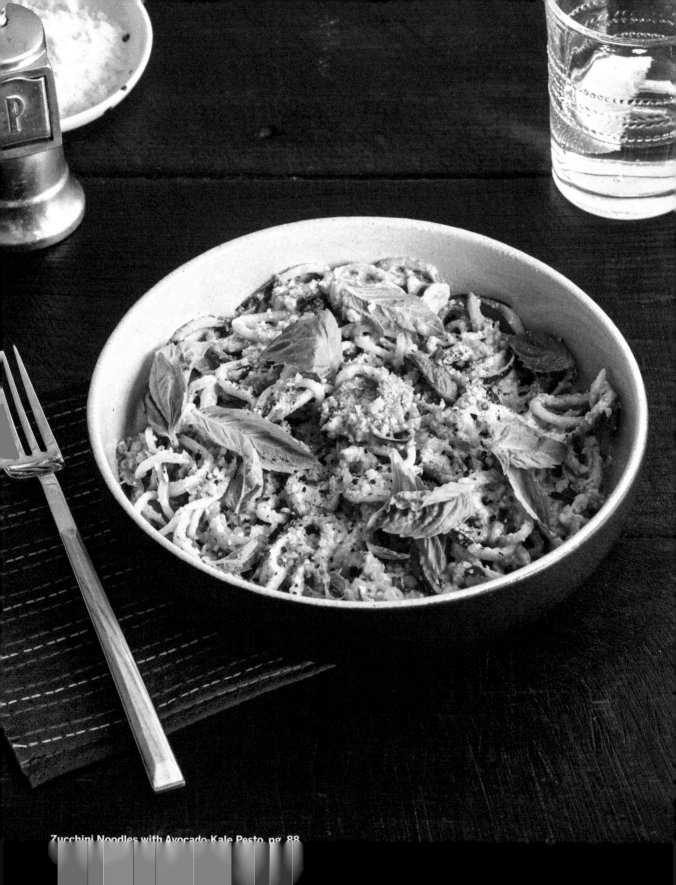

Zucchini Noodles with Avocado-Kale Pesto, pg. 88

CHAPTER THREE

A Weeklong Meal Plan for Every Fast

Changing long-standing eating habits isn't easy. It takes planning, resolve, and a willingness to make sacrifices.

This chapter will help you make these changes. In the pages that follow, you'll find seven-day meal plans for each keto fasting regimen. These plans will put you on autopilot, saving your willpower for the important things in life.

It's not all sacrifice, though. These keto-friendly meals were designed to make your taste buds happy. As an added bonus, everything tastes better after a fast. When you eat less frequently, mealtimes become a real treat.

When you start your keto fasting program, some people will be less supportive than others. Maybe your partner will grumble about you missing family breakfast, or maybe a coworker will needle you to have a piece of cake. *C'mon, one piece won't kill you.*

I've been there. When I radically changed my eating habits in 2011, my fellow employees were less than understanding. Some were mystified, while others loudly mocked my food choices. It wasn't a warm and accepting work environment. I let it get to me.

Today, I'm fortunate enough to engineer my own schedule, but I realize this isn't possible for everyone. You may be stuck with folks who don't get what you're trying to do. In these situations, it pays to remember your priorities: namely, that your health comes first. This is your health journey and nobody else's. Never forget that.

Choosing the Right Fast: The Baby-Step Method

Allow me to introduce the baby-step method of intermittent fasting. The baby-step method is simple: Start with 12/12, and then work your way up the fasting ladder as comfort and schedule permit.

Starting with 12-hour daily fasting:

• gets you a quick win in the fasting game

• is unlikely to cause side effects or discomfort

• still brings metabolic and hormonal benefits

• gives you time to fat-adapt (a must for longer fasts)

Before blowing past 12/12, first think about your priorities. If you need to lose weight, consider creeping toward longer fasts. If you want to build muscle, avoid fasting protocols that restrict calories (such as weekly fasting). And if you're more stressed than a hyperventilated chipmunk, maybe stick with 12/12 for a while. Remember that fasting is a stressor, too.

Fast or Eat Breakfast?

Most fasting regimens don't include a big breakfast, if they include breakfast at all. Is this good or bad?

It depends on your health goals. Skipping breakfast may work for an obese man but not for a normal-weight woman. A 2019 review of the breakfast literature concluded that "the addition of breakfast might not be a good strategy for weight loss." Another study, however, found that female breakfast skippers had higher cortisol and blood pressure than breakfast eaters.

Sleep is another consideration. Eating breakfast (specifically protein) in the morning sets you up for higher levels of melatonin, your sleep hormone, at night. Personally, I like to eat something before noon. I sleep better that way.

You'll have to experiment with skipping breakfast. Maybe it works for you, maybe not.

Daily vs. Weekly Fasts

Both daily and weekly fasts can be beneficial. It's impossible to say which protocol works best for weight loss, disease risk reduction, and so on.

I suggest using two criteria to make your choice: comfort and schedule.

First of all, fasting shouldn't be so uncomfortable that you regret buying a book on fasting. If you're hungry, that's fine. But if you're weak, tired, sleepless, or extremely irritable, you're not doing yourself or those around you any favors by soldiering on.

That's why I recommend the baby-step approach to intermittent fasting. After 12/12, go to 16/8 or 5:2 next. Provided you feel good, feel free to keep baby-stepping up the ladder.

The second criterion is your schedule, especially your social schedule. The more you fast, the less you eat with other humans. If you can't bear the thought of missing half your family dinners, maybe alternate-day fasting isn't for you.

Your work schedule is also relevant. Does your job involve schmoozing clients over lunch? This could cramp your fasting latitude. In the good news column, skipping meals adds hours of focus to your productive day. It's amazing what you can accomplish when you don't have to take time out for eating.

Fast-Specific Meal Plan

In this section you'll find a meal plan for each fasting protocol, complete with keto-friendly recipes from chapters 4 through 10. A few notes before diving in:

- Most meal plans provide between 1,500 and 2,000 calories per day, but you may need to tweak the portions to suit your body. Sustainable weight loss is good, but feeling weak, cold, or sleepless probably means you're not eating enough.

- The meal plans are merely suggestions. Feel free to substitute your own keto-friendly concoctions. (See page 21 for tips on building your keto plate.)

- Don't feel pressure to make every recipe. Leftovers are a big time-saver.

For more details on the following protocols, refer to chapter 1.

Daily Fasts

To practice daily fasting (also called time-restricted feeding), simply eat all your calories within a set time window each day.

12/12 FAST

Do 12/12 right—eat three meals within a 12-hour window—and you shouldn't feel deprived at all. Meanwhile, you'll be supporting sleep, improving insulin function, and priming your fat-burning machinery.

MONDAY
Breakfast: Layered Egg Bake (page 53)
Lunch: Turkey Jalapeño Soup (page 70)
Dinner: Italian Sausage Ratatouille (page 129)

TUESDAY
Breakfast: Lettuce Huevos Rancheros (page 51)
Lunch: Portobello Mushroom Margherita Pizza (page 91)
Dinner: Chicken Thighs in Buttery Lemon Sauce (page 114)

WEDNESDAY
Breakfast: Zucchini Chocolate Bread (page 56)
Lunch: Bean Radish Salad with Sliced Eggs (page 80)
Dinner: Baked Trout with Sesame-Ginger Dressing (page 106)

THURSDAY
Breakfast: Spicy Sausage and Egg–Stuffed Zucchini (page 55)
Lunch: Chilled Avocado-Cilantro Soup with Crab (page 68)
Dinner: Traditional Fried Steak and Eggs (page 133)

FRIDAY
Breakfast: Chicken-Avocado Omelet (page 48)
Lunch: Blue Cheese Bok Choy Salad with Turkey (page 76)
Dinner: Brussels Sprout Ground Pork Hash (page 125)

SATURDAY

Breakfast: Mediterranean Egg Casserole (page 49)
Lunch: Fiery Coconut Noodles (page 90)
Dinner: Sirloin Steak with Creamy Mustard Sauce (page 132)

SUNDAY

Breakfast: Blackberry Cheesecake Smoothie (page 62)
Lunch: Chicken Primavera Sprouts Salad (page 77)
Dinner: Fish Coconut Curry (page 109)

16/8 FAST

For 16/8, simply skip breakfast and eat between the hours of 11 a.m. and 7 p.m. (or some similar time frame). Once you adapt to fasting, 16/8 is easier than it sounds.

MONDAY

Breakfast: FAST
Lunch: Coconut Noodle Crab Salad (page 81)
Dinner: Beef Bacon Burgers (page 130)

TUESDAY

Breakfast: FAST
Lunch: Kale and Chard Shakshuka (page 100)
Dinner: Spicy Pork Lettuce Wraps (page 126)

WEDNESDAY

Breakfast: FAST
Lunch: Bacon Cheeseburger Soup (page 73)
Dinner: Chicken Pot Pie Soup (page 69)

THURSDAY

Breakfast: FAST
Lunch: Fish Avocado Tacos (page 108)
Dinner: "Pasta" Carbonara (page 136)

FRIDAY
Breakfast: FAST
Lunch: Chicken Chow Mein (page 115)
Dinner: Grilled Flank Steak with Bacon Onion Jam (page 134)

SATURDAY
Breakfast: FAST
Lunch: Bacon and Egg Salad (page 79)
Dinner: Jerk Pork Tenderloin (page 123)

SUNDAY
Breakfast: FAST
Lunch: Simple Muffuletta Salad (page 78)
Dinner: Chicken Tenders with Creamy Almond Sauce (page 118)

ONE MEAL A DAY (OMAD)

When you practice OMAD, you eat all your daily calories in one sitting. To prevent nutrient and calorie deficits, scale up your meal size by eating two or three servings of the suggested recipes. If possible, however, avoid stuffing yourself to the gills.

MONDAY
Breakfast: FAST
Lunch: FAST
Dinner: Roasted Red Pepper Konjac Pasta (page 89)

TUESDAY
Breakfast: FAST
Lunch: FAST
Dinner: Chicken Chow Mein (page 115)

WEDNESDAY
Breakfast: FAST
Lunch: FAST
Dinner: Jerk Pork Tenderloin (page 123)

THURSDAY

Breakfast: FAST

Lunch: FAST

Dinner: Shrimp and Sausage Sauté (page 111)

FRIDAY

Breakfast: FAST

Lunch: FAST

Dinner: Rib Eye Steak with Anchovy Compound Butter (page 131)

SATURDAY

Breakfast: FAST

Lunch: FAST

Dinner: Slow Cooker Buffalo Pork with Blue Cheese Dressing (page 127)

SUNDAY

Breakfast: FAST

Lunch: FAST

Dinner: Brown Butter Baked Salmon (page 104)

Weekly Fasts

Next up are your weekly fasting meal plans. These protocols alternate fasting and feeding days.

5:2 FAST

With 5:2 fasting, you pick two days per week (whichever days work best for you) to eat 500 to 700 calories. This tailored meal plan will help.

MONDAY

Breakfast: Traditional Greens-and-Cheese Frittata (page 50)

Lunch: Egg Cauliflower Tikka Masala (page 99)

Dinner: Traditional Fried Steak and Eggs (page 133)

TUESDAY (FAST DAY)
Breakfast: Vegan Bulletproof Coffee Latte (page 150)
Lunch: Mint Strawberry Soda (page 152)
Dinner: Pumpkin Pecan Fat Bombs (eat two) (page 144)

WEDNESDAY
Breakfast: Cinnamon Bun Smoothie (page 60)
Lunch: Fiery Coconut Noodles (page 90)
Dinner: Pork and Mashed Cauliflower Shepherd's Pie (page 122)

THURSDAY (FAST DAY)
Breakfast: Crustless Bacon-Mushroom Quiche (page 52)
Lunch: Lasagna Soup (page 74)
Dinner: Cream-Poached Trout (page 107)

FRIDAY
Breakfast: Smoked Salmon Deviled Eggs (page 140)
Lunch: Jalapeño Lunch Poppers (page 141)
Dinner: Basic Broth (page 66)

SATURDAY
Breakfast: Peanut Butter Coconut Smoothie (page 63)
Lunch: Cauliflower Pumpkin Seed Couscous (page 87)
Dinner: Golden Chicken Asiago (page 116)

SUNDAY
Breakfast: "N'Oatmeal" Coconut Bowl (page 57)
Lunch: Loaded Cauliflower Soup (page 72)
Dinner: California Rolls with Dipping Sauce (page 94)

ALTERNATE-DAY MODIFIED FASTING (ADMF)

ADMF has you eating 25 percent of your normal calories every other day. This plan starts on Monday, but feel free to modify according to your schedule.

MONDAY

Breakfast: Chicken-Avocado Omelet (page 48)
Lunch: Simple Muffuletta Salad (page 78)
Dinner: Baked Nutty Halibut (page 105)

TUESDAY (FAST DAY)

Breakfast: Classic Bulletproof Coffee (page 147)
Lunch: Basic Broth (page 66)
Dinner: Pistachio-Crusted Goat Cheese (page 142)

WEDNESDAY

Breakfast: Nut and Seed Granola (page 58)
Lunch: Shrimp and Avocado Salad (page 82)
Dinner: Frittata with Turkey and Spinach (page 113)

THURSDAY (FAST DAY)

Breakfast: Keto Tea (Latte) (page 149)
Lunch: Cheese-Crusted Portobello Mushrooms (page 143)
Dinner: Buttery Bacon Fat Bombs (eat one) (page 145)

FRIDAY

Breakfast: Mediterranean Egg Casserole (page 49)
Lunch: Bean Radish Salad with Sliced Eggs (page 80)
Dinner: Chile Garlic Sauce Short Ribs (page 135)

SATURDAY (FAST DAY)

Breakfast: Coconut Lime Milkshake (page 153)
Lunch: Chipotle Chocolate Fat Bombs (eat one) (page 146)
Dinner: Basic Broth (page 66)

SUNDAY

Breakfast: Spicy Sausage and Egg–Stuffed Zucchini (page 55)
Lunch: Fiery Coconut Noodles (page 90)
Dinner: Rib Eye Steak with Anchovy Compound Butter (page 131)

ALTERNATE-DAY FASTING (ADF)

At 36 hours between meals, ADF lies on the border between intermittent fasting and extended fasting. If you're following the baby-step method, this is the last rung on the intermittent fasting ladder.

MONDAY

Breakfast: Lime Almond Smoothie (page 59)
Lunch: Double Cheese Soup (page 75)
Dinner: Chili Seafood Stew (page 110)

TUESDAY (FAST DAY)

Breakfast: FAST
Lunch: FAST
Dinner: FAST

WEDNESDAY

Breakfast: Spicy Sausage and Egg–Stuffed Zucchini (page 55)
Lunch: Blue Cheese Bok Choy Salad with Turkey (page 76)
Dinner: Zucchini Noodles with Avocado-Kale Pesto (page 88)

THURSDAY (FAST DAY)

Breakfast: FAST
Lunch: FAST
Dinner: FAST

FRIDAY

Breakfast: Chocolate-Avocado Smoothie (page 61)
Lunch: Kale and Chard Shakshuka (page 100)
Dinner: Turkey Sausage Meatloaf (page 112)

SATURDAY (FAST DAY)

Breakfast: FAST
Lunch: FAST
Dinner: FAST

Breakfast: Lettuce Huevos Rancheros (page 51)
Lunch: Fish Avocado Tacos (page 108)
Dinner: Pork Pumpkin Ragout (page 124)

Thinking Long Term

Most diets fail. After a predictable period of weight loss, the dieter returns to old eating habits. Then the pounds come roaring back.

The problem runs deeper than food. The problem is that diets are temporary by definition, and lasting health improvements aren't achieved by temporary interventions.

What about keto and intermittent fasting? Study after study have shown both programs to promote weight loss, lower insulin, improve fat-burning, and much more. Nonetheless, these studies were conducted over periods of weeks, not years or lifetimes.

Think of keto and intermittent fasting as tools to support your health journey—a power couple that works together to kick-start your metabolism. But keto fasting won't work long term if the rest of your life is out of order. Sure, you might lose weight in the short run, but bad habits have a way of catching up with you.

Getting your health in order means sleeping well, managing stress, eating whole foods, avoiding refined sugar, exercising regularly, getting out into nature, and fostering social connections. The goal isn't to be perfect in all these areas. You won't be. Life is messy, and you're bound to slip up from time to time.

I certainly do. Writing this book, for instance, is a fairly stressful endeavor—but that stress is more than offset by the rewards. The thought of helping people improve their health is a big boost to my energy, happiness, and motivation.

You may get a similar boost just from reading this book. Take advantage of that extra motivation while it's fresh and turn it into action.

Reading this book also means you're the kind of person who cares deeply about your health. I hope you'll maintain this attitude for the rest of your life. It will serve you well.

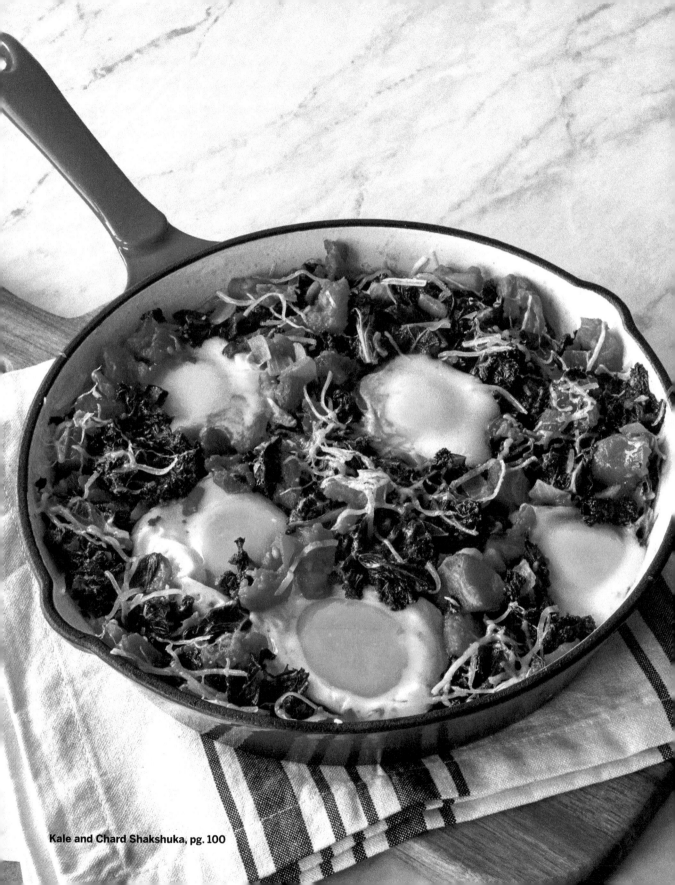

Kale and Chard Shakshuka, pg. 100

PART TWO

Keto Recipes for Your Fast

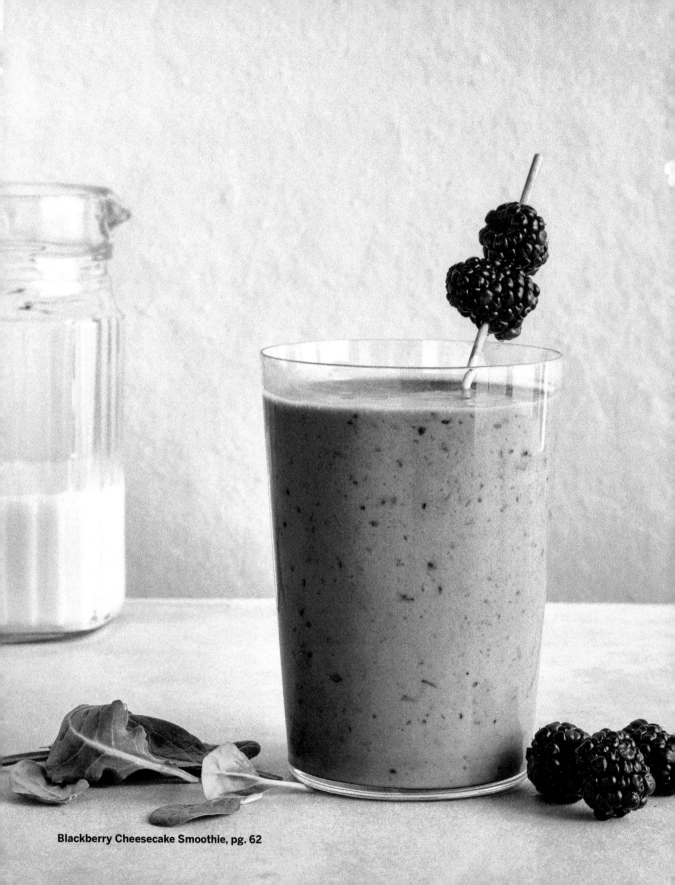

Blackberry Cheesecake Smoothie, pg. 62

Breakfast & Smoothies

Chicken-Avocado Omelet

SERVES 2 / PREP TIME: 15 MINUTES / COOK TIME: 10 MINUTES

1 PAN/1 POT, 30-MINUTE, 500 CALORIES OR FEWER, NUT-FREE

Omelet-making is a valuable skill, and it pays to learn the secrets. The trick to fluffy omelets is to move the beaten eggs continually in your skillet. As the eggs firm up, use the spatula to move the uncooked eggs while continuing to swirl. Say hello to the perfect omelet.

4 large eggs
¼ cup heavy (whipping) cream
2 teaspoons chopped fresh cilantro
Pinch red pepper flakes
2 tablespoons extra-virgin olive oil
½ cup chopped cooked chicken
1 tomato, coarsely chopped
1 avocado, diced
Sea salt
Freshly ground black pepper
¼ cup crumbled feta cheese

1. In a medium bowl, whisk together the eggs, heavy cream, cilantro, and red pepper flakes until well mixed.
2. Heat the olive oil in a large skillet over medium heat.
3. Pour the egg mixture into the skillet and cook until just barely set, lifting the edges with a spatula to let the uncooked egg flow underneath, about 6 minutes.
4. When the egg mixture is firm, scatter the top with the chicken, tomato, and avocado.
5. Season with salt and black pepper.
6. Fold one edge of the omelet over, cut in half, and transfer to 2 plates.
7. Serve topped with the feta cheese.

ADDITION TIP: Double this recipe in an 8-by-8-inch baking dish and a 375°F oven. Arrange the fillings (chicken, avocado, and tomato) in the bottom of the dish and pour the egg mixture over. Top with the cheese. Bake until the egg mixture is cooked through and the top is golden and puffy, about 30 minutes.

PER SERVING: Calories: 200; Total Fat: 17g; Total Carbohydrates: 3g; Net Carbs: 1g; Fiber: 2g; Protein: 9g
MACROS: Fat: 75% / Carbs: 5% / Protein: 20%

Mediterranean Egg Casserole

SERVES 6 / PREP TIME: 15 MINUTES / COOK TIME: 35 MINUTES

500 CALORIES OR FEWER, NUT-FREE, VEGETARIAN

Eggs can be combined with many other ingredients to create savory or sweet dishes. But watch out: When eggs get overcooked, they become rubbery and unpalatable. This is because water in the egg gets squeezed out, the yolk solidifies, and the whites become too tight. The trick is to watch your casserole and use a thermometer (if you have one) to bake the casserole to 160°F.

1 tablespoon extra-virgin olive oil, plus more for greasing
½ onion, chopped
1 red bell pepper, seeded and diced
1 tablespoon minced garlic
8 large eggs
½ cup heavy (whipping) cream
1 cup halved cherry tomatoes
¼ cup sliced black olives
1 cup crumbled goat cheese
2 tablespoons chopped fresh basil, for garnish

1. Preheat the oven to 375°F.
2. Lightly grease a 10-by-10-inch baking dish with olive oil and set aside.
3. Heat 1 tablespoon of olive oil in a large skillet over medium-high heat and sauté the onion, bell pepper, and garlic until softened, about 4 minutes.
4. Transfer the vegetables to the baking dish and spread them out.
5. In a medium bowl, whisk together the eggs and heavy cream until blended and pour over the vegetables in the baking dish.
6. Scatter the tomatoes, olives, and goat cheese over the top of the eggs and bake until the top is puffed and golden brown, about 30 minutes.
7. Serve topped with the basil.

MAKE AHEAD: This recipe freezes beautifully, so portion the cooked casserole when completely cooled and store in the freezer in sealed plastic bags for up to 1 month. Either thaw overnight in the refrigerator or microwave directly from frozen for 4 to 5 minutes.

PER SERVING: Calories: 252; Total Fat: 21g; Total Carbohydrates: 4g; Net Carbs: 3g; Fiber: 1g; Protein: 13g
MACROS: Fat: 73% / Carbs: 7% / Protein: 20%

Traditional Greens-and-Cheese Frittata

SERVES 6 / PREP TIME: 15 MINUTES / COOK TIME: 25 MINUTES

500 CALORIES OR FEWER, NUT-FREE, VEGETARIAN

Eggs are a go-to choice for the keto diet. They naturally have 63 percent fat and 35 percent protein, perfect for reaching your macro goals. Adding kale, sour cream, and cheese in this simple, tasty frittata keeps you in the correct macro range. Whenever possible, purchase organic free-range eggs from a reputable supplier. Not only are the chickens treated better, but the eggs are higher in omega-3 fatty acids and minerals.

1 tablespoon extra-virgin olive oil

12 large eggs

½ cup heavy (whipping) cream

¼ cup sour cream

2 cups frozen chopped kale, thawed with the liquid squeezed out

1 cup shredded Cheddar cheese, divided

¼ teaspoon ground nutmeg

Sea salt

Freshly ground black pepper

1 tablespoon chopped fresh basil, for garnish

1. Preheat the oven to 350°F.
2. Grease a 9-by-13-inch baking dish with the olive oil and set aside.
3. In a medium bowl, whisk together the eggs, the heavy cream, the sour cream, the kale, ½ cup of the Cheddar cheese, and the nutmeg.
4. Season with salt and pepper.
5. Pour the mixture into the baking dish and top with the remaining ½ cup of cheese.
6. Bake until the frittata is puffed and just cooked through, about 25 minutes.
7. Remove from the oven and serve garnished with the basil.

ADDITION TIP: Serve one quarter of this frittata with Bean Radish Salad (page 80) instead of the sliced eggs for a meal with 822 calories. The macros will be Fat: 75% / Carbs: 6% / Protein: 19% with this combination.

PER SERVING: Calories: 332; Total Fat: 28g; Total Carbohydrates: 3g; Net Carbs: 0g; Fiber: 3g; Protein: 19g
MACROS: Fat: 74% / Carbs: 5% / Protein: 21%

Lettuce Huevos Rancheros

SERVES 4 / PREP TIME: 20 MINUTES / COOK TIME: 5 MINUTES

30-MINUTE, 500 CALORIES OR FEWER, NUT-FREE, VEGETARIAN

Huevos rancheros, or "rancher's eggs," is a Mexican breakfast dish beloved by people far and wide. This variation of the spicy dish includes avocado as a pretty topping. Avocado is high in both nutrients and healthy monounsaturated fat. This monounsaturated fat, called oleic acid, helps fill you up and is a fabulous choice for a fasting diet.

1 tablespoon extra-virgin olive oil

8 large eggs

½ jalapeño pepper, finely chopped

8 large Boston lettuce leaves

½ cup salsa

½ cup sour cream

1 cup shredded Cheddar cheese

1 avocado, diced

4 teaspoons chopped fresh cilantro

1. Heat the olive oil in a large skillet over medium-high heat.
2. Add the eggs and jalapeño pepper and scramble until they form light and fluffy curds, about 4 minutes in total. Remove the skillet from the heat.
3. Arrange the lettuce leaves on a serving plate and evenly divide the eggs, salsa, sour cream, Cheddar cheese, avocado, and cilantro among the leaves. Serve.

VARIATION TIP: Chopped cooked chicken or cooked ground beef works well as a protein-packed topping for this filling breakfast wrap. It's good for meeting protein requirements to help you stay lean and strong.

PER SERVING: Calories: 418; Total Fat: 34g; Total Carbohydrates: 9g; Net Carbs: 5g; Fiber: 4g; Protein: 22g
MACROS: Fat: 71% / Carbs: 8% / Protein: 21%

Crustless Bacon-Mushroom Quiche

SERVES 6 / PREP TIME: 10 MINUTES / COOK TIME: 35 MINUTES

500 CALORIES OR FEWER, NUT-FREE

Surprisingly enough, quiche is German in origin, not French. The word "quiche," in fact, comes from the German word for cake: "kuchen." This is a crustless quiche, but if you prefer, it can be baked into a keto-friendly nut-based pie crust. This quiche, you'll be happy to know, is filled with nutritious dark leafy greens. Kale contains compounds with powerful antioxidant effects, plus it's high in calcium, fiber, and vitamins A, C, and K.

1 tablespoon extra-virgin olive oil
8 ounces bacon, chopped
2 cups sliced fresh mushrooms
¼ onion, chopped
1 cup shredded kale or chard
10 large eggs
½ cup heavy (whipping) cream
Sea salt
Freshly ground black pepper
½ cup Swiss or feta cheese
1 teaspoon chopped fresh thyme, for garnish

1. Preheat the oven to 350°F.
2. Heat the olive oil in a large oven-safe skillet over medium-high heat.
3. Fry the bacon until crispy (about 6 minutes), remove from the skillet with a slotted spoon, and place on a paper towel–lined plate.
4. Add the mushrooms and onion to the skillet and sauté until lightly browned, about 5 minutes.
5. Add the kale and sauté until the greens are wilted and most of the liquid is evaporated, about 5 minutes. Return the bacon to the skillet, stirring to combine.
6. In a medium bowl, beat together the eggs and heavy cream and season with salt and pepper.
7. Add the egg mixture to the skillet and cook for 3 to 4 minutes, lifting the edges of the frittata with a spatula so that the uncooked portions flow underneath.
8. Sprinkle the Swiss cheese on top and bake the frittata in the oven until set and lightly browned, about 15 minutes.
9. Remove the frittata from the oven and let stand 5 minutes.
10. Serve immediately, topped with the thyme.

PER SERVING: Calories: 425; Total Fat: 37g; Total Carbohydrates: 4g; Net Carbs: 3g; Fiber: 1g; Protein: 19g
MACROS: Fat: 79% / Carbs: 3% / Protein: 18%

Layered Egg Bake

SERVES 6 / PREP TIME: 15 MINUTES / COOK TIME: 50 MINUTES

NUT-FREE

This layered dish takes time to make, but the finished meal is worth it. To create tasty variations, mix up your vegetable choices or use ground poultry instead of beef. Just hold the quantities and bake time constant to ensure your casserole comes out correctly.

3 tablespoons extra-virgin olive oil, divided, plus more for greasing

8 ounces ground beef

1 cup sliced mushrooms

½ onion, chopped

2 teaspoons minced garlic

2 cups chopped fresh baby spinach

1 zucchini, chopped

1 red bell pepper, chopped

8 large eggs

1 cup heavy (whipping) cream

½ teaspoon salt

½ teaspoon freshly ground black pepper

2 cups shredded Swiss cheese

1. Preheat the oven to 350°F. Lightly grease a 10-by-10-inch casserole dish with olive oil and set aside.

2. Heat 1 tablespoon of olive oil in a large skillet over medium-high heat.

3. Sauté the ground beef until cooked through, breaking it up, about 6 minutes.

4. Transfer the meat to the casserole dish, spreading it out evenly.

5. Place the skillet back on the heat and add 1 tablespoon of oil.

6. Sauté the mushrooms, onion, and garlic until softened, about 5 minutes. Spread the mushroom mixture over the meat.

7. Place the skillet back over the heat and add the remaining 1 tablespoon of oil. Sauté the spinach, zucchini, and bell pepper until softened, about 5 minutes, and then spread it over the mushroom mixture.

8. In a medium bowl, whisk together the eggs, heavy cream, salt, and black pepper and pour the egg mixture over the casserole ingredients. Tap the dish to disperse the mixture to the bottom.

9. Sprinkle the Swiss cheese over the eggs and bake until the eggs are cooked through and the top is golden, about 35 minutes.

CONTINUED ▸

Layered Egg Bake CONTINUED

MAKE AHEAD: This dish can be assembled the night before and baked straight from the refrigerator. (Just increase the final cooking time to 45 to 50 minutes). You can also cook the casserole and freeze it for up to 3 months.

PER SERVING: Calories: 541; Total Fat: 46g; Total Carbohydrates: 7g; Net Carbs: 5g; Fiber: 2g; Protein: 28g
MACROS: Fat: 75% / Carbs: 4% / Protein: 21%

Spicy Sausage and Egg–Stuffed Zucchini

SERVES 4 / PREP TIME: 15 MINUTES / COOK TIME: 35 MINUTES

NUT-FREE

If you wish, use tomatoes, pumpkin, squash, or bell peppers instead of zucchini as vehicles for your filling. Simply scoop out the centers, fill, and bake for the same amount of time in the same temperature oven. Pro tip: Double the filling part of the recipe to create a satisfying meal for extra-hungry guests.

4 medium zucchini

1 tablespoon extra-virgin olive oil, divided

8 ounces Italian sausage (hot or mild)

1 scallion, white and green parts, finely chopped

4 large eggs

½ cup heavy (whipping) cream

Sea salt

Freshly ground black pepper

1 cup shredded sharp Cheddar cheese

1. Preheat the oven to 400°F.
2. Cut a slice off each zucchini lengthwise and scoop out the insides, leaving the outside shell intact. Lightly oil a 9-by-9-inch baking dish with 1 teaspoon of olive oil and set the zucchini in the dish, hollow-side up.
3. Lightly oil the outside of the zucchini with 1 teaspoon of olive oil.
4. Place a small skillet over medium-high heat and add the remaining oil.
5. Sauté the sausage and scallion until the meat is cooked through and browned, about 6 minutes. Then fill each zucchini with equal amounts of the sausage mixture.
6. In a small bowl, whisk the eggs and heavy cream and season with salt and pepper.
7. Fill each zucchini with equal amounts of the egg mixture and top with the Cheddar cheese.
8. Bake until the eggs are firm, the zucchini is softened, and the cheese is lightly browned, about 30 minutes.

MAKE AHEAD: Make the recipe, place the stuffed vegetables in the baking dish, and store covered in the refrigerator overnight. Bake the stuffed vegetables straight out of the refrigerator for 35 to 40 minutes.

PER SERVING: Calories: 544; Total Fat: 47g; Total Carbohydrates: 7g; Net Carbs: 5g; Fiber: 2g; Protein: 26g
MACROS: Fat: 75% / Carbs: 5% / Protein: 20%

Zucchini Chocolate Bread

SERVES 8 / PREP TIME: 15 MINUTES / COOK TIME: 1 HOUR

500 CALORIES OR FEWER, DAIRY-FREE, VEGETARIAN

Let's be honest. This chocolatey bread is pretty much dessert for breakfast. When eating one meal a day, you might combine a couple slices of this bread with an omelet or frittata to reach 900 to 1,000 calories. This recipe uses zucchini, which can aid the digestive process following a fast.

½ cup coconut oil, melted, plus
  more for greasing the
  loaf pan
1 cup almond flour
1 cup granulated erythritol
½ cup coconut flour
¼ cup cocoa powder
1½ teaspoons baking powder
1 teaspoon ground cinnamon
½ teaspoon baking soda
¼ teaspoon salt
4 large eggs
2 teaspoons vanilla extract
2 cups finely grated zucchini

1. Preheat the oven to 350°F.
2. Lightly grease a 9-by-4-inch loaf pan with coconut oil and set aside.
3. In a large bowl, stir together the almond flour, erythritol, coconut flour, cocoa powder, baking powder, cinnamon, baking soda, and salt until well blended.
4. In a medium bowl, whisk together the eggs, coconut oil, and vanilla until mixed.
5. Add the wet ingredients to the dry ingredients and stir until just combined.
6. Stir in the zucchini.
7. Spoon the batter into the prepared loaf pan and bake until a knife inserted in the center comes out clean, about 1 hour.
8. Let the bread cool completely.
9. Store wrapped in the refrigerator for up to 4 days or in the freezer for up to 1 month.

CRAVING TIP: Made with shredded zucchini and unsweetened cocoa powder, this bread is not overly sweet but will still satisfy your sweet tooth. Also, the fiber in the loaf will keep you feeling full longer.

PER SERVING: Calories: 286; Total Fat: 22g; Total Carbohydrates: 14g; Net Carbs: 6g; Fiber: 8g; Protein: 8g; Erythritol Carbs: 24mg
MACROS: Fat: 67% / Carbs: 19% / Protein: 14%

"N'Oatmeal" Coconut Bowl

SERVES 4 / PREP TIME: 10 MINUTES / COOK TIME: 10 MINUTES

1 PAN/1 POT, 30-MINUTE, 500 CALORIES OR FEWER, DAIRY-FREE, VEGAN

Oatmeal is a classic, wholesome breakfast dish that sticks to the ribs, but it's not keto friendly. That's where this coconut-based oatmeal comes in. The combination of nuts, seeds, and sweetener can be adjusted according to your preference, but keep in the almond flour and coconut to maintain the cooked cereal texture.

1 cup coconut milk, plus more for serving if necessary

½ cup shredded unsweetened coconut

¼ cup almond flour

¼ cup chopped pecans

¼ cup granulated erythritol

2 tablespoons hemp hearts

2 scoops vanilla protein powder

½ teaspoon ground cinnamon

¼ teaspoon ground nutmeg

1. In a medium saucepan over low heat, stir together the coconut milk, shredded coconut, almond flour, pecans, erythritol, hemp hearts, protein powder, cinnamon, and nutmeg.

2. Cook, stirring occasionally, until the mixture has heated through and thickened, 8 to 10 minutes. Serve.

MAKE AHEAD: This recipe is mostly dry ingredients, so you can double them and store in a container with a lid for later. Simply use ¾ cup of dry ingredients and ¼ cup coconut or nut milk per portion.

PER SERVING: Calories: 447; Total Fat: 35g; Total Carbohydrates: 12g; Net Carbs: 4g; Fiber: 8g; Protein: 21g; Erythritol Carbs: 12g
MACROS: Fat: 70% / Carbs: 10% / Protein: 20%

Nut and Seed Granola

SERVES 4 / PREP TIME: 10 MINUTES / COOK TIME: 1 HOUR

DAIRY-FREE, VEGAN

I bet you didn't think you could have granola on keto, did you? Granola contains nuts, seeds, and other healthy fats that can be enjoyed with a splash of nut milk or as a topping. This recipe contains flaxseed, a superfood packed with omega-3 fatty acids, fiber, antioxidants, and B vitamins. Enjoy.

1 cup sliced almonds

½ cup shredded unsweetened coconut

¼ cup chopped pecans

¼ cup hazelnuts

½ cup raw pumpkin seeds

¼ cup hemp hearts

¼ cup whole flaxseed

¼ cup melted coconut oil

½ teaspoon ground cinnamon

1. Preheat the oven to 250°F and line a baking sheet with parchment paper.
2. In a large bowl, toss together the almonds, shredded coconut, pecans, hazelnuts, pumpkin seeds, hemp hearts, and flaxseed until mixed.
3. Add the coconut oil and cinnamon to the nut mixture and stir until very well coated.
4. Spread the granola on the baking sheet and bake, stirring occasionally, until crunchy and golden brown, about 1 hour.
5. Let the granola cool on the sheet, and then break it up and store it in an airtight container in the refrigerator or freezer for up to 3 months.

MAKE AHEAD: Granola can be enjoyed on its own, as a topping, or as a base for parfaits. You can multiply this recipe and store it (in sealed bags) in the freezer for up to 3 months. It's perfect for healthy snacking.

PER SERVING (¾ CUP): Calories: 596; Total Fat: 56g; Total Carbohydrates: 14g; Net Carbs: 5g; Fiber: 9g; Protein: 17g
MACROS: Fat: 80% / Carbs: 8% / Protein: 12%

Lime Almond Smoothie

SERVES 2 / PREP TIME: 5 MINUTES

1 PAN/1 POT, 30-MINUTE, VEGETARIAN

Lime has an evocative flavor, conjuring visions of sandy beaches and fruity drinks adorned with parasols. Add coconut oil and almonds to create this sublime smoothie packing 535 calories of healthy fats and protein. And if you want to boost protein, throw in a tablespoon of hemp hearts or a half cup of silken tofu.

1 cup unsweetened
  almond milk

½ cup heavy (whipping) cream

¼ cup raw almonds

¼ cup freshly squeezed
  lime juice

2 scoops vanilla
  protein powder

1 tablespoon coconut oil

1 tablespoon granulated
  erythritol

1 teaspoon freshly grated
  lime zest

1. Combine the almond milk, heavy cream, almonds, lime juice, protein powder, coconut oil, erythritol, and lime zest in a blender and blend until smooth.

2. Pour into 2 glasses and serve immediately.

VARIATION TIP: Try using a citrus-flavored protein powder—orange creamsicle or mango perhaps—to pair nicely with the lime flavor of this smoothie.

PER SERVING: Calories: 535; Total Fat: 39g; Total Carbohydrates: 16g; Net Carbs: 9g; Fiber: 7g; Protein: 30g; Erythritol Carbs: 6g
MACROS: Fat: 66% / Carbs: 12% / Protein: 22%

Cinnamon Bun Smoothie

SERVES 2 / PREP TIME: 5 MINUTES

1 PAN/1 POT, 30-MINUTE, 500 CALORIES OR FEWER, DAIRY-FREE, VEGETARIAN

Cinnamon evokes memories of holidays, warmth, and family that wrap around you like cozy blankets. And guess what: Cinnamon adds not just flavor but also vitamin K, calcium, iron, and manganese to this heavenly smoothie. This popular spice can also help stabilize blood sugar, which comes in handy for staying in ketosis. Make sure your ground cinnamon is less than six months old. This will ensure potency.

1 cup unsweetened
  almond milk
½ cup coconut milk
1 avocado, diced
1 scoop vanilla protein powder
1 tablespoon granulated
  erythritol
1 teaspoon ground cinnamon
½ teaspoon vanilla extract
2 tablespoons chopped
  pecans, for garnish

1. Combine the almond milk, coconut milk, avocado, protein powder, erythritol, cinnamon, and vanilla extract in a blender and blend until smooth.

2. Pour into 2 glasses and serve immediately, topped with the pecans.

ADDITION TIP: To increase the fat grams in this rich smoothie, swap out the coconut milk for an equivalent portion of heavy cream. This increases calories to 536 per serving and changes the macros to Fat: 68% / Carbs: 12% / Protein: 20%.

PER SERVING: Calories: 446; Total Fat: 30g; Total Carbohydrates: 17g; Net Carbs: 7g; Fiber: 10g; Protein: 27g; Erythritol Carbs: 6g
MACROS: Fat: 61% / Carbs: 15% / Protein: 24%

Chocolate-Avocado Smoothie

SERVES 2 / PREP TIME: 10 MINUTES

1 PAN/1 POT, 30-MINUTE, 500 CALORIES OR FEWER, DAIRY-FREE, VEGETARIAN

Dark chocolate is keto-approved, in moderate amounts at least. So go ahead and indulge in this rich almond milkshake packed with minerals such as magnesium, iron, copper, and manganese. Cocoa supports a healthy cardiovascular system and may help reduce cognitive decline. Plus the protein powder doubles up the rich flavor and adds necessary texture.

½ cup coconut milk

½ cup unsweetened almond milk

1 avocado, diced

¼ cup cocoa powder

¼ cup ground flaxseed

1½ scoops chocolate protein powder

2 tablespoons granulated erythritol

¼ teaspoon ground cinnamon

4 ice cubes

1. Combine the coconut milk, almond milk, avocado, cocoa powder, flaxseed, protein powder, erythritol, and cinnamon in a blender and process until very smooth.
2. Add the ice to the blender and process again until very thick and smooth.
3. Pour into 2 glasses and serve.

CRAVING TIP: People love chocolate. Movies have been made about this obsession. If chocolate is your weakness, this milkshake-like creation will satisfy you completely.

PER SERVING: Calories: 456; Total Fat: 32g; Total Carbohydrates: 17g; Net Carbs: 5g; Fiber: 12g; Protein: 25g; Erythritol Carbs: 12g
MACROS: Fat: 64% / Carbs: 14% / Protein: 22%

Blackberry Cheesecake Smoothie

SERVES 2 / PREP TIME: 10 MINUTES

1 PAN/1 POT, 30-MINUTE, 500 CALORIES OR FEWER, VEGETARIAN

Blackberries might not be your first choice of berry, but perhaps that should change. Blackberries are extremely rich in fiber (about five grams in two-thirds of a cup) as well as vitamins C and K. Blackberry seeds are also a good source of protein, omega-3 fatty acids, and fiber. Because of the health benefits of the seeds and other berry components, whole berries are preferable to smooth strained purée for your recipes.

1 cup unsweetened almond milk
⅔ cup cream cheese
½ cup blackberries
½ cup shredded fresh baby spinach
1 scoop vanilla protein powder
1 tablespoon granulated erythritol

1. Combine the almond milk, cream cheese, blackberries, spinach, protein powder, and erythritol in a blender and blend until smooth.
2. Pour into 2 glasses and serve immediately.

ADDITION TIP: This is not an overly sweet smoothie. The blackberries add a certain tartness, so drinking a large amount won't be overwhelming. You could use this entire recipe as one serving and enjoy a quick 754-calorie meal.

PER SERVING: Calories: 377; Total Fat: 29g; Total Carbohydrates: 10g; Net Carbs: 5g; Fiber: 5g; Protein: 19g; Erythritol Carbs: 6g
MACROS: Fat: 70% / Carbs: 20% / Protein: 10%

Peanut Butter Coconut Smoothie

SERVES 2 / PREP TIME: 10 MINUTES

1 PAN/1 POT, 30-MINUTE, 500 CALORIES OR FEWER, DAIRY-FREE, VEGETARIAN

What could be more decadent than a peanut butter milkshake? If you consume the "N'Oatmeal" Coconut Bowl (page 57) and this smoothie, you will have a satisfying 840-calorie combination that will get you close to your daily needs. For an exciting candy-bar-like smoothie, swap out the vanilla protein powder for chocolate protein powder and add a couple of tablespoons of low-carb chocolate chips as a garnish.

½ cup coconut milk
½ cup unsweetened
  almond milk
1 cup cooked cauliflower
2 tablespoons natural
  peanut butter
1 scoop vanilla protein powder
3 ice cubes

1. Combine the coconut milk, almond milk, cauliflower, peanut butter, and protein powder in a blender and blend until smooth.

2. Add the ice and blend until smooth.

3. Pour into 2 glasses and serve immediately.

MAKE AHEAD: Cooked cauliflower is a perfect way to add fiber and other nutrients to your meal. Steam or blanch an entire head and store the vegetable in handy 1-cup portions in the refrigerator for up to 5 days or in the freezer for up to 3 months.

PER SERVING: Calories: 393; Total Fat: 29g; Total Carbohydrates: 13g; Net Carbs: 6g; Fiber: 7g; Protein: 20g
MACROS: Fat: 66% / Carbs: 14% / Protein: 20%

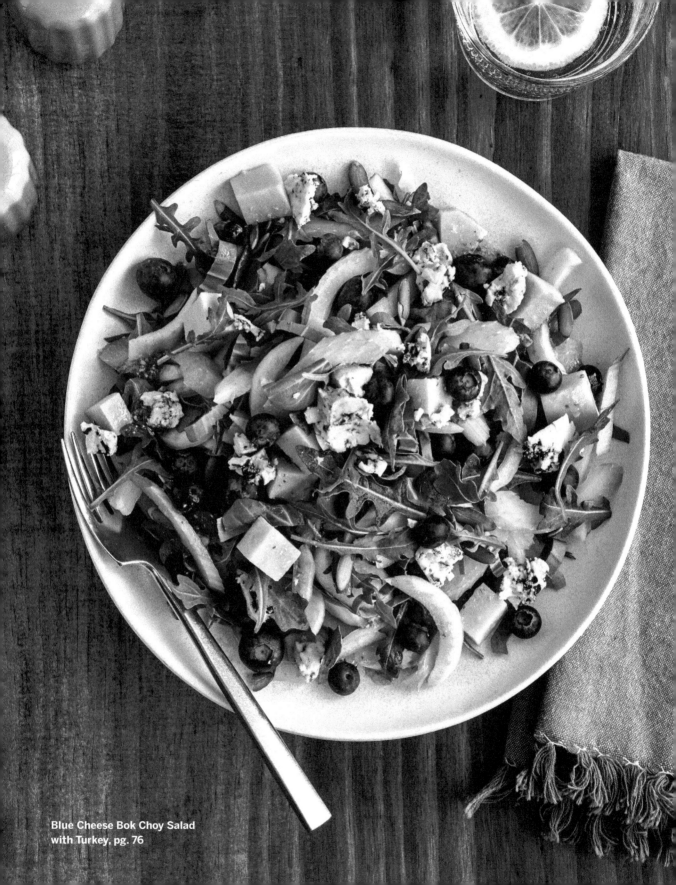

Blue Cheese Bok Choy Salad
with Turkey, pg. 76

Soups & Salads

Basic Broth

MAKES 8 CUPS / PREP TIME: 15 MINUTES / COOK TIME: 2 TO 3 HOURS

500 CALORIES OR FEWER, ALLERGEN-FREE, VEGAN

Broth takes a little effort to make, but it's well worth it. After all, you can never be sure about the additives and ingredients in store-bought soups. For a set-it-and-forget-it method, use a slow cooker instead of a pot. Simply toss the ingredients inside the slow cooker and fill with water until 1½ inches from the top. Cover and cook the broth on low for 10 to 12 hours, strain out the solids, cool, and store. Now you have a simple option for fasting days or a delicious base for any soup.

4 garlic cloves, crushed

3 celery stalks with greens, roughly chopped

2 carrots, roughly chopped

1 onion, peeled and quartered

½ cup chopped fresh parsley

4 thyme sprigs

2 bay leaves

½ teaspoon peppercorns

½ teaspoon salt

8 cups water

1. Combine the garlic, celery, carrots, onion, parsley, thyme, bay leaves, peppercorns, and salt in a large stockpot.
2. Add the water, cover, and bring to a boil.
3. Reduce the heat to low and simmer gently for 2 to 3 hours.
4. Strain the broth through a fine-mesh sieve and discard the solids.
5. Store the broth in sealed containers in the refrigerator for up to 5 days or in the freezer for up to 1 month.

BEEF BROTH VARIATION: Add 2 to 3 pounds of beef bones (beef marrow, knuckle bones, ribs, and any other bones) and 2 tablespoons of apple cider vinegar in step 1 of the Basic Broth recipe and enough water to cover the extra ingredients. Simmer, scooping off any accumulating foam, for 6 to 7 hours. (Don't scoop if using a slow cooker.) Strain the broth through a fine-mesh sieve, discarding the solids. After cooling, store the broth in sealed containers in the refrigerator for up to 1 week or in the freezer for up to 3 months. Makes 8 cups.

CHICKEN BROTH VARIATION: Add 2 chicken carcasses and 2 tablespoons of apple cider vinegar in step 1 of the Basic Broth recipe and enough water to cover the extra ingredients. Simmer, scooping off any accumulating foam, for 4 to 5 hours. (Don't scoop if using a slow cooker.) Strain the broth through a fine-mesh sieve, discarding the solids. After cooling, store the broth in sealed containers in the refrigerator for up to 1 week or in the freezer for up to 3 months. Makes 8 cups.

FISH BROTH VARIATION: Add 3 to 4 pounds of fish bones and heads to the Basic Broth recipe and enough water to cover the extra ingredients. Simmer for 1 hour, and then strain the broth through a fine-mesh sieve, discarding the solids. After cooling, store the broth in sealed containers in the refrigerator for up to 1 week or in the freezer for up to 3 months. Makes 8 cups.

VEGETABLE BROTH PER SERVING (1 CUP): Calories: 24; Total Fat: 0g; Total Carbohydrates: 4g; Net Carbs: 4g; Fiber: 0g; Protein: 2g
MACROS: Fat: 2% / Carbs: 66% / Protein: 32%
BEEF BROTH PER SERVING (1 CUP): Calories: 42; Total Fat: 1g; Total Carbohydrates: 0g; Net Carbs: 0g; Fiber: 0g; Protein: 8g
MACROS: Fat: 20% / Carbs: 4% / Protein: 76%
CHICKEN BROTH PER SERVING (1 CUP): Calories: 38; Total Fat: 0g; Total Carbohydrates: 0g; Net Carbs: 0g; Fiber: 0g; Protein: 9g
MACROS: Fat: 5% / Carbs: 1% / Protein: 94%
FISH BROTH PER SERVING (1 CUP): Calories: 34; Total Fat: 1g; Total Carbohydrates: g; Net Carbs: g; Fiber: g; Protein: 7g
MACROS: Fat: 26% / Carbs: 2% / Protein: 72%

Chilled Avocado-Cilantro Soup with Crab

SERVES 6 / PREP TIME: 15 MINUTES

30-MINUTE, 500 CALORIES OR FEWER, NUT-FREE

Chilled soups are popular in many cultures across the world. Avocado makes the perfect base ingredient for this cold soup—so lusciously creamy, so thick when puréed. Then there's the rich crab. If fresh crab isn't available, pick up some frozen crabmeat. Just give it time to thaw and squeeze out any excess liquid to prevent overdiluting the soup.

2 avocados, diced

2 cups coconut water

1 cup heavy (whipping) cream

1 English cucumber, cut into chunks

1 cup watercress

½ onion, diced

½ cup roughly chopped fresh cilantro

Juice of 1 lime

2 teaspoons ground cumin

Sea salt

Freshly ground black pepper

1 pound cooked crabmeat

1. Combine the avocados, coconut water, heavy cream, cucumber, watercress, onion, cilantro, lime juice, and cumin in a blender and purée until very smooth.
2. Season with salt and pepper.
3. Serve topped with the crabmeat.

MAKE AHEAD: When making this soup ahead, add a little extra lime juice to prevent the avocado from turning brown and oxidizing. Only add the crab when you're ready to serve.

PER SERVING: Calories: 296; Total Fat: 23g; Total Carbohydrates: 9g; Net Carbs: 5g; Fiber: 4g; Protein: 17g
MACROS: Fat: 67% / Carbs: 10% / Protein: 23%

Chicken Pot Pie Soup

SERVES 6 / PREP TIME: 20 MINUTES / COOK TIME: 35 MINUTES

500 CALORIES OR FEWER, NUT-FREE

Chunks of tender chicken, oodles of chopped vegetables, and pinches of fragrant herbs combine with creamy, cheesy broth to create this mouthwatering soup. For a real treat, spoon it into an oven-safe bowl, top with Swiss or mozzarella cheese, broil until melted and golden brown, and serve. This charming presentation adds just over 100 calories and 8 grams of fat and protein per serving.

2 tablespoons extra-virgin olive oil, divided

1 pound skinless chicken breast, cut into ½-inch chunks

1 onion, chopped

1 cup quartered mushrooms

2 celery stalks, chopped

2 carrots, diced

1 tablespoon minced garlic

5 cups low-sodium chicken broth

1 cup heavy (whipping) cream

¼ cup cream cheese

1 cup chopped green beans

1 tablespoon chopped fresh thyme

Salt

Freshly ground black pepper

1. Heat 1 tablespoon of olive oil in a large stockpot over medium-high heat and sauté the chicken breast until just cooked through, about 10 minutes.

2. With a slotted spoon, remove the chicken to a plate and set aside.

3. Add the remaining 1 tablespoon of oil and sauté the onion, mushrooms, celery, carrots, and garlic until softened, 6 to 7 minutes.

4. Stir in the chicken broth and reserved chicken and bring the soup to a boil. Reduce the heat to low and simmer until the vegetables are tender, about 15 minutes.

5. Stir in the heavy cream, cream cheese, green beans, and thyme and simmer for 3 minutes.

6. Season with salt and pepper and serve hot.

MAKE AHEAD: If you wish to freeze this soup, hold off on adding the heavy cream during preparation. This will prevent the soup from splitting when thawed. While reheating the frozen soup, stir in the cream, and then serve.

PER SERVING: Calories: 336; Total Fat: 26g; Total Carbohydrates: 7g; Net Carbs: 5g; Fiber: 2g; Protein: 20g
MACROS: Fat: 70% / Carbs: 5% / Protein: 25%

Turkey Jalapeño Soup

SERVES 6 / PREP TIME: 15 MINUTES / COOK TIME: 20 MINUTES

1 PAN/1 POT, ALLERGEN-FREE

If you enjoy simple hearty soups, this recipe is for you. The jalapeño pepper adds a kick, plus there are onions, carrots, and cabbage for bulk, fiber, and flavor. All that fiber, by the way, helps fill you up. Make sure you follow the directions carefully and add the cabbage at the end. If cabbage simmers too long, it becomes slimy and malodorous.

3 tablespoons coconut oil
1 onion, chopped
1 jalapeño pepper, chopped
1 tablespoon minced garlic
1 tablespoon peeled grated fresh ginger
12 ounces cooked diced turkey
1 carrot, diced
6 cups low-sodium chicken broth
2 cups coconut milk
Zest and juice of 1 lime
1 cup shredded cabbage
2 tablespoons chopped fresh cilantro, for garnish

1. Heat the coconut oil in a large stockpot over medium-high heat.
2. Sauté the onion, jalapeño, garlic, and ginger until softened, about 5 minutes.
3. Add the turkey, carrot, chicken broth, coconut milk, and lime juice and zest to the stockpot.
4. Bring the soup to a boil; then reduce the heat to low and simmer until the vegetables are tender, about 10 minutes.
5. Add the cabbage and simmer for 5 minutes.
6. Serve topped with the cilantro.

MAKE AHEAD: This soup can be doubled and frozen with no loss of taste or texture. Portion the soup into single servings in containers or freezer bags, and thaw when ready to eat.

PER SERVING: Calories: 508; Total Fat: 40g; Total Carbohydrates: 13g; Net Carbs: 11g; Fiber: 2g; Protein: 25g
MACROS: Fat: 70% / Carbs: 9% / Protein: 21%

Reuben Soup

SERVES 4 / PREP TIME: 15 MINUTES / COOK TIME: 20 MINUTES

1 PAN/1 POT, 500 CALORIES OR FEWER, NUT-FREE

This unusual soup, based on the classic sandwich, might become your new favorite. It's salty, spicy, tart, and sweet—and parsley adds an unexpected earthy flavor. Parsley is not just a topping; it also contains folate and several flavonoids, such as luteolin, quercetin, and kaempferol, that help protect cells from oxidative stress.

3 tablespoons extra-virgin olive oil

1 onion, chopped

2 celery stalks, chopped

1 tablespoon minced garlic

6 cups low-sodium beef broth

12 ounces corned beef, chopped

2 cups sauerkraut

2 tablespoons hot mustard

½ teaspoon caraway seeds

1½ cups shredded Swiss cheese

2 tablespoons chopped fresh parsley, for garnish

1. Heat the olive oil in a large stockpot over medium-high heat and sauté the onion, celery, and garlic until softened, about 5 minutes.
2. Stir in the beef broth, corned beef, sauerkraut, mustard, and caraway seeds and bring to a boil.
3. Reduce the heat to low and simmer until the vegetables are tender, about 15 minutes.
4. Serve topped with the Swiss cheese and parsley.

CRAVING TIP: Reuben sandwiches are packed with layers of meat, tart sauerkraut, and melted Swiss cheese. Yum. The only element missing here is the bread, but caraway seeds evoke the taste of rye, so that should help.

PER SERVING: Calories: 493; Total Fat: 38g; Total Carbohydrates: 9g; Net Carbs: 6g; Fiber: 3g; Protein: 30g
MACROS: Fat: 68% / Carbs: 7% / Protein: 25%

Loaded Cauliflower Soup

SERVES 6 / PREP TIME: 15 MINUTES / COOK TIME: 25 MINUTES

1 PAN/1 POT, 500 CALORIES OR FEWER, NUT-FREE

This loaded soup is . . . well . . . *loaded* with vegetables, cream, bacon, and cheese. Every spoonful is filled with flavor. Instead of leaving the cauliflower florets whole, you can also purée the soup in a food processor or blender before adding the cream. If you like crispy bacon, don't add it directly to the soup, but instead use it as a topping along with the cheese and scallions.

3 tablespoons extra-virgin
   olive oil
1 onion, chopped
2 teaspoons minced garlic
6 cups chopped cauliflower
6 cups low-sodium
   chicken broth
2 cups heavy (whipping) cream
1 cup cooked chopped bacon
1 teaspoon ground nutmeg
Sea salt
Freshly ground black pepper
1 cup shredded
   Cheddar cheese
1 scallion, white and green
   parts, chopped

1. Heat the olive oil in a large stockpot over medium-high heat.
2. Sauté the onion and garlic until softened, about 3 minutes.
3. Add the cauliflower and chicken broth to the stockpot.
4. Bring the soup to a boil, then reduce the heat to low and simmer until the vegetables are tender, about 20 minutes.
5. Stir in the heavy cream, bacon, and nutmeg.
6. Season with salt and pepper and serve topped with the Cheddar cheese and scallions.

CRAVING TIP: This soup should satisfy a craving for loaded baked potatoes because it contains similar flavors. Add 1 tablespoon of sour cream per bowl to complete this classic culinary combination.

PER SERVING: Calories: 429; Total Fat: 36g; Total Carbohydrates: 9g; Net Carbs: 6g; Fiber: 3g; Protein: 19g
MACROS: Fat: 74% / Carbs: 7% / Protein: 19%

Bacon Cheeseburger Soup

SERVES 6 / PREP TIME: 15 MINUTES / COOK TIME: 35 MINUTES

1 PAN/1 POT, NUT-FREE

Dill pickle in your soup? Yes, the briny flavor complements the bacon, Cheddar, and beef broth in this recipe. Feel free to also add mustard. This tastes great the next day, too.

3 tablespoons extra-virgin olive oil, divided

8 ounces ground beef

1 onion, chopped

2 celery stalks, chopped

1 carrot, shredded

1 tablespoon minced garlic

4 cups low-sodium beef broth

1 (15-ounce) can low-sodium diced tomatoes

1 cup heavy (whipping) cream

1 cup shredded sharp Cheddar cheese

8 cooked bacon slices, chopped

2 tablespoons chopped dill pickles, for garnish

2 tablespoons chopped fresh parsley, for garnish

1. Heat 2 tablespoons of olive oil in a large stockpot over medium-high heat.
2. Sauté the ground beef until browned and cooked through, about 6 minutes. With a slotted spoon, remove to a plate.
3. Add the remaining 1 tablespoon of oil and sauté the onion, celery, carrot, and garlic until softened, about 6 minutes.
4. Stir in the beef broth, tomatoes, and reserved beef and bring the soup to a boil.
5. Reduce the heat to low and simmer until the vegetables are tender, about 15 minutes.
6. Add the heavy cream, Cheddar cheese, and bacon and stir until the cheese is melted, about 3 minutes.
7. Serve topped with the chopped pickle and parsley.

ADDITION TIP: If you are following a single-meal fasting plan, double the portion to get 1,072 calories. Rest assured, your macros will stay in order.

PER SERVING: Calories: 536; Total Fat: 44g; Total Carbohydrates: 9g; Net Carbs: 2g; Fiber: 7g; Protein: 26g
MACROS: Fat: 74% / Carbs: 6% / Protein: 20%

Lasagna Soup

SERVES 6 / PREP TIME: 15 MINUTES / COOK TIME: 35 MINUTES

500 CALORIES OR FEWER, NUT-FREE

This flavorful soup features vegetables, tomatoes, ground beef, herbs, and lots of melty mozzarella cheese. The macros are perfectly balanced in this dish, so feel free to multiply your servings and use during OMAD or 16/8 protocols (see chapter 3).

3 tablespoons extra-virgin olive oil, divided

12 ounces ground beef

1 onion, chopped

1 green bell pepper, diced

1 tablespoon minced garlic

4 cups low-sodium beef broth

1 (15-ounce) can diced tomatoes, undrained

1 zucchini, diced

1 cup fresh baby spinach

1 tablespoon chopped fresh basil

1 tablespoon chopped fresh oregano

1 cup shredded mozzarella

1. Heat 1 tablespoon of olive oil in a large stockpot over medium-high heat and sauté the ground beef until browned and cooked through, about 6 minutes.

2. With a slotted spoon, remove the beef to a plate and set aside.

3. Add the remaining 2 tablespoons of oil to the stockpot and sauté the onion, bell pepper, and garlic until softened, about 4 minutes.

4. Stir in the beef broth, tomatoes with their juice, zucchini, and reserved beef and bring to a boil.

5. Reduce the heat to low and simmer until the vegetables are tender, about 20 minutes.

6. Stir in the spinach, basil, and oregano and simmer for 2 minutes.

7. Remove from the heat and stir in the mozzarella. Serve hot.

ADDITION TIP: Stir in a quarter cup of soft goat cheese or cream cheese (per serving) to create a richer soup with about 200 more calories. This tweak adds 20 grams of fat and 3 grams of protein.

PER SERVING: Calories: 321; Total Fat: 25g; Total Carbohydrates: 8g; Net Carbs: 5g; Fiber: 3g; Protein: 16g
MACROS: Fat: 70% / Carbs: 10% / Protein: 20%

Double Cheese Soup

SERVES 6 / PREP TIME: 15 MINUTES / COOK TIME: 30 MINUTES

1 PAN/1 POT, NUT-FREE

Cheese lovers will adore this creamy creation. You might think you'll only taste cream cheese and Cheddar, but wait until the garlic, onion, and celery hit your palate. Celery, by the way, adds vitamins A, B, and C as well as potassium, calcium, and iron to the dish. Potassium is crucial for maintaining healthy blood pressure, among other functions.

2 tablespoons extra-virgin olive oil
1 onion, chopped
2 celery stalks, chopped
1 carrot, chopped
1 teaspoon minced garlic
5 cups low-sodium chicken broth
1 cup coconut milk
⅛ teaspoon red pepper flakes
2 cups shredded sharp Cheddar cheese
6 ounces cream cheese, cubed
Salt
Freshly ground black pepper
8 cooked bacon slices, chopped

1. Heat the olive oil in a large stockpot over medium-high heat and sauté the onion, celery, carrot, and garlic until softened, about 6 minutes.
2. Stir in the chicken broth, coconut milk, and red pepper flakes and bring the soup to a boil.
3. Reduce the heat to low and simmer until the vegetables are tender, about 15 minutes.
4. Stir in the Cheddar and cream cheeses and continue cooking until the cheeses are melted and the soup is smooth, about 4 minutes.
5. Season with salt and pepper.
6. Serve topped with the bacon.

SUBSTITUTION TIP: For a vegetarian creation, swap the chicken broth for vegetable broth and omit the bacon. To maintain your macros, add a couple scoops of unflavored vegan protein powder in step 4.

PER SERVING: Calories: 551; Total Fat: 47g; Total Carbohydrates: 8g; Net Carbs: 6g; Fiber: 2g; Protein: 24g
MACROS: Fat: 76% / Carbs: 6% / Protein: 18%

Blue Cheese Bok Choy Salad with Turkey

SERVES 6 / PREP TIME: 25 MINUTES

30-MINUTE, 500 CALORIES OR FEWER

Crisp, juicy bok choy stands out among the blue cheese, turkey, and blueberries that round out this salad. Bok choy is high in calcium, potassium, folate, and vitamins A, C, and K, so it helps support immunity, bone health, and more. Take extra care when washing bok choy. The curved stem at the bottom is usually filled with dirt, and you don't want that in your salad.

FOR THE VINAIGRETTE

⅓ cup macadamia nut oil
¼ cup apple cider vinegar
1 tablespoon grainy Dijon mustard
2 teaspoons granulated erythritol
1 teaspoon minced garlic
Sea salt
Freshly ground black pepper

FOR THE SALAD

6 cups shredded baby bok choy
2 cups arugula
2 celery stalks, cut into thin slices
4 ounces chopped cooked turkey breast
½ cup fresh blueberries
¼ cup pumpkin seeds
1 cup crumbled blue cheese

TO MAKE THE VINAIGRETTE

1. In a small bowl, whisk together the macadamia nut oil, apple cider vinegar, mustard, erythritol, and garlic until well blended.
2. Season with salt and pepper and set aside.

TO MAKE THE SALAD

1. In a large bowl, toss together the bok choy, arugula, celery, turkey, blueberries, and pumpkin seeds with half the vinaigrette.
2. Arrange the salads on 6 plates and evenly divide the blue cheese among them.
3. Drizzle with the remaining vinaigrette and serve.

ADDITION TIP: Double the serving size in order to double the calories to 574 to suit your specific fasting plan (see chapter 3). But no matter the portion size, the macros will stay perfect.

PER SERVING: Calories: 287; Total Fat: 23g; Total Carbohydrates: 5g; Net Carbs: 3g; Fiber: 2g; Protein: 14g; Erythritol Carbs: 1g
MACROS: Fat: 73% / Carbs: 7% / Protein: 20%

Chicken Primavera Sprouts Salad

SERVES 4 / PREP TIME: 30 MINUTES

30-MINUTE, 500 CALORIES OR FEWER, DAIRY-FREE

Don't let the fear of shredding vegetables stop you from making this salad; it won't take as long as you think. To cut down your shredding or dicing prep time, pick up a mandoline at your local kitchen store. This tool cuts prep time in half for most recipes, but please be careful because the blades are incredibly sharp.

½ cup avocado oil mayonnaise

2 tablespoons basil pesto

2 cups bean sprouts

2 cups shredded red cabbage

1 cup shredded broccoli

1 carrot, shredded

1 cup shredded cooked chicken

½ cup roasted pumpkin seeds

1. In a small bowl, stir together the mayonnaise and pesto until well blended. Set aside.

2. In a large bowl, toss together the sprouts, cabbage, broccoli, carrot, chicken, and pumpkin seeds until well mixed.

3. Add the dressing and toss to coat. Serve.

SUBSTITUTION TIP: Replace the pesto with 2 tablespoons apple cider vinegar and 1 teaspoon granulated erythritol for a traditional coleslaw dressing. This change will reduce the fat in the recipe to 30 grams per serving and change the macros to Fat: 69% / Carbs: 9% / Protein: 22%.

PER SERVING: Calories: 420; Total Fat: 33g; Total Carbohydrates: 12g; Net Carbs: 9g; Fiber: 3g; Protein: 21g
MACROS: Fat: 70% / Carbs: 10% / Protein: 20%

Simple Muffuletta Salad

SERVES 4 / PREP TIME: 25 MINUTES

30-MINUTE, NUT-FREE

Originally created by Italian immigrants, the muffuletta is a meat and cheese–packed sandwich made on a whole loaf of bread. This salad skips the bread, of course, but still is flavored with traditional olives, garlic, and fresh herbs.

FOR THE DRESSING

½ cup extra-virgin olive oil
3 tablespoons
  balsamic vinegar
1 teaspoon chopped
  fresh oregano
½ teaspoon minced garlic
¼ teaspoon minced fresh basil
Sea salt
Freshly ground black pepper

FOR THE SALAD

4 cups chopped
  romaine lettuce
1 red bell pepper, chopped
½ red onion, chopped
1 cup giardiniera salad, drained
  and chopped
4 ounces sliced provolone
  cheese, chopped
3 ounces sliced spicy
  capicola, chopped
3 ounces sliced genoa
  salami, chopped
3 ounces sliced
  mortadella, chopped
3 ounces sliced
  prosciutto, chopped
½ cup sliced black olives
¼ cup shredded
  mozzarella cheese

TO MAKE THE DRESSING

1. In a small bowl, whisk together the olive oil, balsamic vinegar, oregano, garlic, and basil until well combined.
2. Season with salt and pepper and set aside.

TO MAKE THE SALAD

1. In a large bowl, toss together the lettuce, bell pepper, onion, giardiniera salad, provolone cheese, capicola, salami, mortadella, and prosciutto.
2. Add the dressing and toss to coat.
3. Serve topped with the olives and mozzarella cheese.

ADDITION TIP: This is a full-meal salad, completely packed with meats, cheeses, and vegetables. It will fill you up. If you are eating a single meal, add an after-meal cup of Classic Bulletproof Coffee (page 147) or Keto Tea (Latte) (page 149) to boost the calories to over 1000.

PER SERVING: Calories: 627; Total Fat: 51g; Total Carbohydrates: 12g; Net Carbs: 9g; Fiber: 3g; Protein: 30g
MACROS: Fat: 73% / Carbs: 7% / Protein: 20%

Bacon and Egg Salad

SERVES 6 / PREP TIME: 20 MINUTES

1 PAN/1 POT, 30-MINUTE, 500 CALORIES OR FEWER, NUT-FREE

Bacon and eggs are a staple keto meal. If you add a bacon fat–based dressing, cheese, and crisp romaine, you have a culinary sensation. To avoid overcooking the hardboiled eggs, start them in a pot of cold water (about 1 inch above the eggs), bring the water to a boil, remove the pot from the heat, and let the eggs stand, covered, for 12 minutes. Cool them in cold running water and store in the refrigerator until needed.

4 tablespoons melted bacon fat or extra-virgin olive oil

2 tablespoons apple cider vinegar

Freshly ground black pepper

8 cups chopped romaine lettuce

8 cooked bacon slices, chopped

¼ cup grated Parmesan cheese

4 large hardboiled eggs, chopped

1. In a large bowl, whisk the bacon fat and apple cider vinegar until emulsified. Season with pepper.
2. Add the lettuce, bacon, and Parmesan cheese to the bowl and toss to coat.
3. Top with the hardboiled eggs and serve.

SUBSTITUTION TIP: For a creamier creation, replace the fat-based dressing with a Caesar dressing. The fat grams will be slightly lower, but the macros will still be keto.

PER SERVING: Calories: 297; Total Fat: 25g; Total Carbohydrates: 4g; Net Carbs: 4g; Fiber: 0g; Protein: 16g
MACROS: Fat: 75% / Carbs: 3% / Protein: 22%

Bean Radish Salad with Sliced Eggs

SERVES 4 / PREP TIME: 20 MINUTES

30-MINUTE, 500 CALORIES OR FEWER, DAIRY-FREE, NUT-FREE, VEGETARIAN

Radishes are an underused vegetable. This is a shame because radishes are divine in both color and texture. Radishes grow in a wide range of flavors, from searing hot to slightly peppery. Pick up a bunch of radishes so that you can enjoy the greens sautéed in a stir-fry or, if they are young and tender, in a salad. Radishes contain compounds called anthocyanins that have been shown in animal studies to improve heart health and reduce cancer risk.

FOR THE DRESSING

¼ cup extra-virgin olive oil

2 tablespoons apple cider vinegar

1 teaspoon chopped fresh thyme

1 teaspoon granulated erythritol

Sea salt

Freshly ground black pepper

FOR THE SALAD

4 cups mixed baby greens

2 cups green beans, cut into 1-inch pieces

2 cups quartered radishes

1 English cucumber, diced

4 large hardboiled eggs, sliced

½ cup roasted pumpkin seeds

2 tablespoons hemp hearts

TO MAKE THE DRESSING

1. In a small bowl, whisk together the olive oil, apple cider vinegar, thyme, and erythritol until well combined.

2. Season with salt and pepper and set aside.

TO MAKE THE SALAD

1. In a large bowl, toss together the baby greens, green beans, radishes, and cucumber.

2. Add the dressing and toss to coat.

3. Top with the egg slices, pumpkin seeds, and hemp hearts and serve.

SUBSTITUTION TIP: Replace the eggs with 4 ounces cooked chicken, turkey, beef, or fish for a filling meal. This change will increase the protein per serving by about 3 grams.

PER SERVING: Calories: 396; Total Fat: 32g; Total Carbohydrates: 10g; Net Carbs: 6g; Fiber: 4g; Protein: 17g; Erythritol Carbs: 1g
MACROS: Fat: 72% / Carbs: 10% / Protein: 18%

Coconut Noodle Crab Salad

SERVES 4 / PREP TIME: 30 MINUTES

500 CALORIES OR FEWER, DAIRY-FREE, NUT-FREE

Festive zucchini noodles, bright carrot and red pepper, and deep green cilantro dance in a creamy citrus-infused sauce in this visually stunning salad. Cilantro has a pungent, assertive flavor and adds vitamins A, C, and K as well as potassium, calcium, iron, and manganese to the dish.

FOR THE DRESSING

½ cup coconut milk
2 tablespoons coconut oil
Juice and zest of 1 lime
1 tablespoon erythritol
1 teaspoon coconut aminos
½ teaspoon minced garlic
½ teaspoon grated
   fresh ginger

FOR THE NOODLES

4 cups spiralized zucchini
1 red bell pepper, julienned
1 carrot, shredded
1 jalapeño pepper, seeded
   and minced
2 scallions, white and green
   parts, thinly sliced
8 ounces crabmeat
½ cup shredded
   unsweetened coconut
2 tablespoons chopped fresh
   cilantro, for garnish

TO MAKE THE DRESSING

In a small bowl, whisk together the coconut milk, coconut oil, lime juice and zest, erythritol, coconut aminos, garlic, and ginger until well blended. Set aside.

TO MAKE THE NOODLES

1. In a large bowl, toss together the zucchini, bell pepper, carrot, jalapeño, and scallions until well mixed.
2. Add the dressing and toss to coat.
3. Arrange the salad on 4 plates and evenly divide the crab and shredded coconut among them.
4. Serve topped with the cilantro.

CRAVING TIP: Healthy fats (such as the coconut milk and coconut oil in the dressing) help fill you up better than carbs. More fat means less snacking.

PER SERVING: Calories: 314; Total Fat: 24g; Total Carbohydrates: 12g; Net Carbs: 7g; Fiber: 5g; Protein: 17g; Erythritol Carbs: 3g
MACROS: Fat: 66% / Carbs: 14% / Protein: 20%

Shrimp and Avocado Salad

SERVES 4 / PREP TIME: 20 MINUTES / COOK TIME: 5 MINUTES

30-MINUTE, 500 CALORIES OR FEWER, DAIRY-FREE, NUT-FREE

Some salads are complex, while others are beautifully simple. This salad is the latter. Green pastels, deep emerald, and the pink of shrimp make a pleasing feast for the eyes. Shrimp is not just attractive, it's also a superb source of vitamin B_{12}, vitamin D, iron, and selenium. Frozen cooked shrimp works well with this dish if you like your shrimp cold.

2 tablespoons coconut oil

12 ounces (31–35 count) shrimp, peeled, deveined, and tails removed

8 cups baby mixed greens (spinach, kale, arugula)

1 cup snow peas, stringed

½ English cucumber, diced

½ cup Sesame-Ginger Dressing (page 159), divided

1 avocado, diced

2 tablespoons chopped fresh cilantro, for garnish

1. Heat the coconut oil in a large skillet over medium-high heat and sauté the shrimp until pink and just cooked through, 4 to 5 minutes.
2. Remove the skillet from the heat and set the shrimp aside.
3. In a large bowl, toss the baby greens, snow peas, and cucumber with half the dressing and arrange the mixture on 4 plates.
4. Top the salads with the shrimp and avocado and drizzle the salads with the remaining dressing.
5. Serve topped with the cilantro.

SUBSTITUTION TIP: If you have a shellfish allergy, omit shrimp and use chicken or turkey instead. The poultry adds 2 grams of protein per serving.

PER SERVING: Calories: 395; Total Fat: 30g; Total Carbohydrates: 14g; Net Carbs: 6g; Fiber: 8g; Protein: 19g
MACROS: Fat: 69% / Carbs: 11% / Protein: 20%

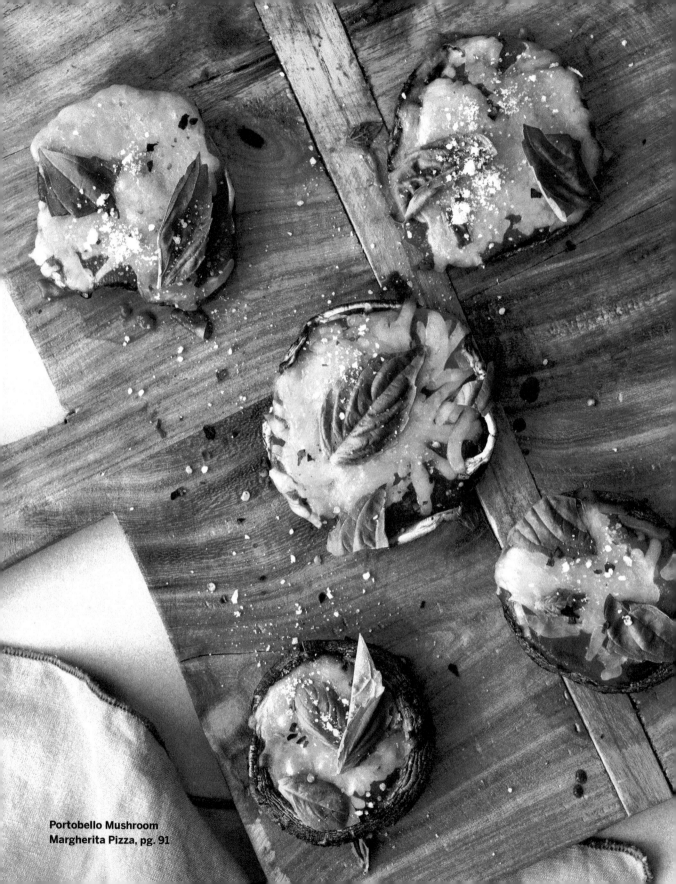

**Portobello Mushroom
Margherita Pizza, pg. 91**

CHAPTER SIX

Vegetarian & Vegan Mains

Spicy Cheese-and-Olive Squares

SERVES 8 / PREP TIME: 15 MINUTES / COOK TIME: 30 MINUTES

500 CALORIES OR FEWER, VEGETARIAN

Jalapeño pepper heats up these cheesy squares, perfect for spicy-food lovers. Add briny black olives and you have a truly complex delight. Black olives, by the way, are packed with heart-friendly monounsaturated fats, vitamin E, and iron. Whenever possible, purchase whole olives and pit them yourself. Pre-sliced olives are mushy in texture and often too salty for the refined palate.

2 tablespoons extra-virgin olive oil, plus more for greasing the baking dish

1 onion, chopped

1 jalapeño pepper, finely chopped

2 teaspoons minced garlic

8 large eggs

1 cup shredded Cheddar cheese

½ cup cream cheese, at room temperature

½ cup sliced black ripe olives

½ cup halved cherry tomatoes

¼ cup ground almonds

2 tablespoons finely chopped fresh cilantro

Sea salt

Freshly ground black pepper

1. Preheat the oven to 325°F. Lightly grease an 8-by-8-inch baking dish with olive oil and set aside.
2. Heat the oil in a medium skillet over medium-high heat.
3. Sauté the onion, jalapeño, and garlic until softened, about 5 minutes. Then remove from the heat and transfer to a large bowl.
4. Add the eggs, Cheddar cheese, cream cheese, olives, tomatoes, ground almonds, and cilantro to the bowl and whisk until well combined. Season with salt and pepper.
5. Pour the mixture into the baking dish and bake until a toothpick inserted into the center comes out clean, about 25 minutes.
6. Allow to cool for 10 minutes and cut into 8 squares. Serve.

ADDITION TIP: Depending on your calorie needs, cut these nutritious squares into whatever portion size suits you. Four servings would be 506 calories per serving, and two servings are 1,012 calories each.

PER SERVING: Calories: 253; Total Fat: 21g; Total Carbohydrates: 4g; Net Carbs: 3g; Fiber: 1g; Protein: 12g
MACROS: Fat: 75% / Carbs: 5% / Protein: 20%

Cauliflower Pumpkin Seed Couscous

SERVES 3 / PREP TIME: 15 MINUTES / COOK TIME: 10 MINUTES

30-MINUTE, ALLERGEN-FREE, VEGAN/VEGETARIAN

Cauliflower couscous has a fluffy texture and soaks up the spices just like real couscous. Cauliflower is not only versatile for making keto-friendly pastas and rice, but it is also high in fiber, manganese, and vitamins C and K to support digestive and heart health.

1 head cauliflower, cut into florets
¼ cup extra-virgin olive oil
1 red bell pepper, finely chopped
1 teaspoon ground coriander
½ teaspoon ground cinnamon
¼ teaspoon paprika
½ cup roasted pumpkin seeds
3 tablespoons hemp hearts
1 scallion, green part only, finely chopped

1. In a food processor, pulse the cauliflower until it is very finely chopped, similar to rice.
2. Heat the olive oil in a large skillet over medium-high heat and add the cauliflower, bell pepper, coriander, cinnamon, and paprika.
3. Sauté until the cauliflower is fluffy and tender, stirring frequently, about 7 minutes.
4. Stir in the pumpkin seeds and hemp hearts.
5. Serve topped with the scallion.

MAKE AHEAD: Store uncooked cauliflower in sealed plastic bags for up to 4 days in the refrigerator and up to 2 months in the freezer. You can also cook cauliflower rice directly from the freezer, no thawing required.

PER SERVING: Calories: 506; Total Fat: 40g; Total Carbohydrates: 15g; Net Carbs: 9g; Fiber: 6g; Protein: 26g
MACROS: Fat: 70% / Carbs: 11% / Protein: 19%

Zucchini Noodles with Avocado-Kale Pesto

SERVES 4 / PREP TIME: 15 MINUTES / COOK TIME: 5 MINUTES

1 PAN/1 POT, 5-INGREDIENT, 30-MINUTE, 500 CALORIES OR FEWER, VEGETARIAN

Simple is best when you need a quick, satisfying meal. What's simpler than vegetable noodles tossed with flavor-packed pesto? You'll find spiralized zucchini in most grocery stores, and it keeps fresh for nearly a week in the refrigerator. Zucchini is rich in antioxidants such as beta-carotene and lutein, and it combines well with the avocado-rich pesto because the monounsaturated fats in avocado increase the absorption of fat-soluble beta-carotene.

1 tablespoon extra-virgin olive oil

4 large zucchini, spiralized (or about 2 pounds if pre-packaged)

¾ cup Avocado-Kale Pesto (page 164)

1 cup grated Parmesan cheese

1 tablespoon chopped fresh basil, for garnish

1. Heat the olive oil in a large skillet over medium heat and sauté the zucchini noodles until just heated through, about 4 minutes.
2. Add the pesto to the skillet and toss to coat.
3. Serve topped with the Parmesan cheese and basil.

SUBSTITUTION TIP: If you wish, use basil pesto or sun-dried tomato pesto in place of the Avocado-Kale Pesto. Most pesto is high in fat and moderately high in protein, so you should be fine on macros.

PER SERVING: Calories: 297; Total Fat: 23g; Total Carbohydrates: 9g; Net Carbs: 5g; Fiber: 4g; Protein: 15g
MACROS: Fat: 70% / Carbs: 10% / Protein: 20%

Roasted Red Pepper Konjac Pasta

SERVE 3 / PREP TIME: 15 MINUTES / COOK TIME: 35 MINUTES

NUT-FREE, VEGETARIAN

Konjac (or shirataki) noodles add almost no carbs to your pasta recipes. Shirataki means "white waterfall" in Japanese, and you'll know why when you toss them into your skillet. The noodles, by the way, are made of a special fiber called glucomannan that comes from the konjac plant. Pro tip: You'll need to rinse off the liquid these noodles come packaged in. Don't worry if they're a little slimy.

4 red bell peppers, halved and seeded
½ onion, cut into eighths
3 garlic cloves, crushed
¼ cup extra-virgin olive oil
1 cup heavy (whipping) cream
Sea salt
Freshly ground black pepper
1 pound konjac noodles
1 cup shredded Parmesan cheese

1. Preheat the oven to 425°F. Line a baking sheet with aluminum foil and set aside.
2. In a large bowl, toss the bell peppers, onion, garlic, and olive oil until well mixed.
3. Transfer the oiled vegetables to the prepared baking sheet and spread them out in a single layer. Roast until very tender and lightly charred, about 20 minutes.
4. Remove the vegetables from the oven and let cool for 10 minutes; then peel the skin off the peppers. Transfer the vegetables to a food processor and purée until smooth.
5. Transfer the sauce to a large saucepan and cook over medium heat until heated through, about 5 minutes.
6. Stir in the heavy cream and season with salt and pepper.
7. While the sauce is cooking, place a medium saucepan filled with water over high heat and bring to a boil.
8. Rinse and drain the konjac noodles and add them to the boiling water. Boil them for 5 minutes; then drain and add to the sauce.
9. Serve topped with the Parmesan cheese.

SUBSTITUTION TIP: If you can't find konjac noodles, you can also use spiralized zucchini or cauliflower rice as the base for the sauce. The sauce is also lovely spooned over chicken or fish and adds a nice hit of protein to your meals.

PER SERVING: Calories: 523; Total Fat: 47g; Total Carbohydrates: 13g; Net Carbs: 8g; Fiber: 5g; Protein: 15g
MACROS: Fat: 78% / Carbs: 10% / Protein: 12%

Fiery Coconut Noodles

SERVES 4 / PREP TIME: 20 MINUTES / COOK TIME: 15 MINUTES

500 CALORIES OR FEWER, DAIRY-FREE, VEGAN

These noodles are savory and warming, thanks in large part to the ginger in this recipe. Ginger has been used for centuries to treat inflammation, headaches, and nausea. Fresh ginger is best to ensure potency, so keep some fresh ginger root around at all times. If you find young ginger roots in an Asian market, you'll notice that the skin is extra thin and doesn't need to be peeled before consuming.

FOR THE SAUCE

½ cup coconut milk
½ cup natural peanut butter
2 tablespoons peeled grated fresh ginger
1 tablespoon coconut aminos
2 teaspoons minced garlic
1 teaspoon granulated erythritol
Juice from 1 lime
Pinch red pepper flakes

FOR THE NOODLES

1 tablespoon coconut oil
2 cups bean sprouts
1 red bell pepper, julienned
1 cup julienned bok choy
1 cup shredded red cabbage
1 cup julienned fresh coconut (optional)
2 scallions, white and green parts, thinly sliced
2 tablespoons chopped fresh cilantro, for garnish

TO MAKE THE SAUCE

1. Whisk together the coconut milk, peanut butter, ginger, coconut aminos, garlic, erythritol, lime juice, and red pepper flakes in a medium saucepan over medium heat.
2. Bring the sauce to a boil; then reduce the heat to low and simmer for about 4 minutes to blend the flavors.
3. Remove the sauce from the heat and set aside.

TO MAKE THE NOODLES

1. Heat the coconut oil in a large skillet over medium-high heat.
2. Sauté the bean sprouts, bell pepper, bok choy, cabbage, fresh coconut (if using), and scallions until they are tender-crisp, 7 to 8 minutes.
3. Stir in the sauce and toss to coat.
4. Serve topped with the cilantro.

CRAVING TIP: The sauce and noodle ingredients in this recipe are hot, sweet, and salty. In other words, this baby will satisfy many cravings. If you prefer a sweeter dish, simply use more erythritol.

PER SERVING: Calories: 376; Total Fat: 28g; Total Carbohydrates: 15g; Net Carbs: 10g; Fiber: 5g; Protein: 16g; Erythritol Carbs: 1g
MACROS: Fat: 68% / Carbs: 15% / Protein: 17%

Portobello Mushroom Margherita Pizza

SERVES 6 / PREP TIME: 15 MINUTES / COOK TIME: 10 MINUTES

5-INGREDIENT, 30-MINUTE, 500 CALORIES OR FEWER, NUT-FREE, VEGETARIAN

Portobello mushrooms have a meaty texture that soaks up spices, herbs, and other flavorings like a sponge. It's no wonder they're a main course in many vegan and vegetarian restaurants. Mushrooms are a rare vegetable source of vitamin D and also contain high levels of potassium. The cheese and olive oil (the fats) in this recipe help you absorb that all-important vitamin D.

½ cup extra-virgin olive oil

1 teaspoon minced garlic

6 large portobello mushrooms, stems removed

1 cup low-carb tomato sauce

2 cups shredded mozzarella cheese

2 tablespoons chopped fresh basil, for garnish

1. Preheat the oven to broil. Line a baking sheet with aluminum foil and set aside.
2. In a medium bowl, stir together the olive oil and garlic; then add the mushrooms to the bowl. Rub the oil all over the mushrooms and place them gill-side down on the prepared baking sheet.
3. Broil the mushrooms until they are tender, turning once, about 4 minutes in total.
4. Remove the baking sheet from the oven and evenly divide the tomato sauce among the mushroom caps, spreading it on the gill side. Then top with the mozzarella cheese.
5. Broil the mushrooms until the cheese is melted and bubbly, 1 to 2 minutes.
6. Serve topped with the basil.

VARIATION TIP: If you're not vegetarian, pepperoni, Italian sausage, and prosciutto are delectable additions to these hearty pizzas. Meat will add protein and a few grams of fat to the dish.

PER SERVING: Calories: 325; Total Fat: 25g; Total Carbohydrates: 9g; Net Carbs: 6g; Fiber: 3g; Protein: 16g
MACROS: Fat: 70% / Carbs: 10% / Protein: 20%

Wild Mushroom Tofu Ragù

SERVES 4 / PREP TIME: 15 MINUTES / COOK TIME: 25 MINUTES

1 PAN/1 POT, 500 CALORIES OR FEWER, NUT-FREE, VEGETARIAN

Mushrooms have an earthy taste that complements the heavy cream, garlic, and thyme in this stew. Herbs might seem insignificant, but these superfood plants are staples in many international cuisines. Thyme, for instance, is high in volatile oils and flavonoids as well as vitamin K and iron. Be generous with your thyme shaker, and your body will thank you.

3 tablespoons extra-virgin olive oil

2 zucchini, diced

1 onion, chopped

1 tablespoon minced garlic

1 pound assorted wild mushrooms, sliced

8 ounces extra-firm tofu, pressed

1 cup heavy (whipping) cream

½ cup low-sodium vegetable broth

2 teaspoons chopped fresh thyme

Sea salt

Freshly ground black pepper

1. Heat the olive oil in a large skillet over medium-high heat.
2. Sauté the zucchini, onion, and garlic until tender, about 6 minutes.
3. Stir in the mushrooms and tofu and sauté until the liquid purges and the mushrooms caramelize, about 10 minutes.
4. Stir in the heavy cream, vegetable broth, and thyme and bring the ragù to a boil.
5. Reduce the heat to low and simmer until the sauce thickens, about 6 minutes.
6. Season with salt and pepper and serve.

SUBSTITUTION TIP: For a vegan-friendly option, swap the heavy cream for coconut milk (same amount) and add a scoop of vegan protein powder. This will change the calories to 395 per serving and the macros to Fat: 71% / Carbs: 9% / Protein: 20%.

PER SERVING: Calories: 456; Total Fat: 40g; Total Carbohydrates: 9g; Net Carbs: 6g; Fiber: 3g; Protein: 15g
MACROS: Fat: 78% / Carbs: 8% / Protein: 14%

Vegetable Avocado Stew

SERVES 8 / PREP TIME: 15 MINUTES / COOK TIME: 20 MINUTES

1 PAN/1 POT, 500 CALORIES OR FEWER, NUT-FREE, VEGETARIAN

This avocado-based stew has a subtle flavor and sits nicely in your stomach. Combining it with the Pork and Mashed Cauliflower Shepherd's Pie (page 122) would net you 625 calories in total. You could also add a couple cups of cooked chicken or turkey if you're okay with animal products.

2 tablespoons extra-virgin olive oil

1 onion, chopped

1 red bell pepper, diced

1 tablespoon peeled grated fresh ginger

2 teaspoons minced garlic

2 cups low-sodium vegetable broth

2 scoops unflavored vegan protein powder

2 tablespoons curry powder

2 cups heavy (whipping) cream

1 cup cauliflower florets

1 cup broccoli florets

1 avocado, diced

1 tablespoon chopped fresh parsley, for garnish

1. Heat the olive oil in a large stockpot over medium-high heat.
2. Sauté the onion, bell pepper, ginger, and garlic until softened, about 5 minutes.
3. Stir the vegetable broth, protein powder, and curry powder into the pot.
4. Bring the mixture to a boil; then reduce the heat to low and simmer for 5 minutes. Stir in the heavy cream, cauliflower, and broccoli and simmer for 10 minutes more.
5. Serve topped with the avocado and parsley.

ADDITION TIP: Double the portion size to increase the calories to 678 per serving. You can add a generous scoop, about ¼ cup, of Greek yogurt to increase the protein grams by 2 to 3 grams.

PER SERVING: Calories: 339; Total Fat: 27g; Total Carbohydrates: 12g; Net Carbs: 6g; Fiber: 6g; Protein: 12g
MACROS: Fat: 72% / Carbs: 13% / Protein: 15%

California Rolls with Dipping Sauce

SERVES 4 / PREP TIME: 30 MINUTES / COOK TIME: 5 MINUTES

500 CALORIES OR FEWER, ALLERGEN-FREE, VEGAN

Sushi looks complicated to make, but once you master the art of nori rolling, you'll be serving it regularly. To simplify your prep, pick up a sushi rolling mat. You'll use this mat as a base to make your rolls.

3 tablespoons extra-virgin olive oil
1 carrot, shredded
1 cup shredded baby bok choy
1 red bell pepper, julienned
1 cup julienned snow peas
1 cup bean sprouts
3 tablespoons sesame seeds
4 nori sheets
1 avocado, thinly sliced
½ cup Sesame-Ginger Dressing (page 159)

1. Heat the olive oil in a large skillet over medium-high heat.
2. Sauté the carrot, bok choy, bell pepper, and snow peas until tender-crisp, about 4 minutes.
3. Remove the skillet from the heat and transfer the vegetables to a medium bowl.
4. Add the bean sprouts and sesame seeds to the bowl and toss to mix.
5. Lay a sheet of nori shiny-side down on a clean work surface.
6. Spread a quarter of the vegetables all along the edge closest to you and top with a quarter of the avocado.
7. Roll the sushi away from you to create a tight sushi roll, taking care to wet the far edge so that it sticks.
8. Set aside and complete the other three rolls.
9. Cut each sushi roll into 5 pieces with a serrated knife and serve with the Sesame-Ginger Dressing.

VARIATION TIP: Add shredded chicken, crab, or shrimp to increase the protein in the dish. Four ounces of chicken adds 9 grams of protein, 1 gram of fat, and 46 calories per portion. The macros become: Fat: 74% / Carbs: 10% / Protein: 16%.

PER SERVING: Calories: 404; Total Fat: 36g; Total Carbohydrates: 12g; Net Carbs: 6g; Fiber: 6g; Protein: 8g
MACROS: Fat: 80% / Carbs: 12% / Protein: 8%

Sesame Tofu Broccoli Fried Rice

SERVES 4 / PREP TIME: 20 MINUTES / COOK TIME: 20 MINUTES

500 CALORIES OR FEWER, DAIRY-FREE, NUT-FREE, VEGAN

Most low-carb diets extol the virtues of cauliflower rice, but broccoli rice is just as good. Broccoli might not look like white rice, but the texture is similar, especially when fried until tender-crisp. Broccoli contains a compound called sulforaphane, which has powerful anticancer properties, so whip up a batch of this broccoli rice and get chomping. Broccoli also contains high levels of calcium and folate—both essential nutrients for bone health, nervous system function, and more.

3 tablespoons coconut oil, divided

1 pound extra-firm tofu, pressed

1 tablespoon sesame oil

2 heads broccoli, finely chopped

2 celery stalks, thinly sliced

1 red bell pepper, thinly sliced

1 tablespoon minced garlic

1 teaspoon peeled grated fresh ginger

2 tablespoons coconut aminos

1 scallion, white and green parts, thinly sliced on the diagonal

2 tablespoons sesame seeds, for garnish

1. Heat 2 tablespoons of coconut oil in a large skillet or wok over medium-high heat.
2. Sauté the tofu until crispy and browned, about 5 minutes. With a slotted spoon, remove to a plate.
3. Add the remaining 1 tablespoon of coconut oil and the sesame oil to the skillet and sauté the broccoli, celery, bell pepper, garlic, and ginger until the vegetables are tender-crisp, 10 to 12 minutes.
4. Stir in the reserved tofu, coconut aminos, and scallion and sauté for 1 minute more.
5. Serve topped with the sesame seeds.

SUBSTITUTION OR VARIATION TIP: Replace the broccoli with cauliflower (equal amounts) as preference and availability dictate.

PER SERVING: Calories: 328; Total Fat: 24g; Total Carbohydrates: 12g; Net Carbs: 8g; Fiber: 4g; Protein: 16g
MACROS: Fat: 66% / Carbs: 12% / Protein: 22%

Creamy Veggie Tofu Stroganoff

SERVES 4 / PREP TIME: 15 MINUTES / COOK TIME: 20 MINUTES

1 PAN/1 POT, 500 CALORIES OR FEWER, NUT-FREE, VEGETARIAN

Stroganoff is a Russian dish that was, it's believed, originally created by a French chef. This hearty meal usually features beef strips, mushrooms, cream, and loads of paprika. Here we use tofu instead of beef. Paprika is a red spice with a spicy, smoky flavor made from dried red bell peppers and chiles. Paprika contains multiple antioxidant compounds that may improve eye health.

¼ cup extra-virgin olive oil

1 onion, chopped

4 cups sliced white
   mushrooms

1 tablespoon minced garlic

8 ounces extra-firm tofu,
   pressed then cut into
   1-inch cubes

2 cups low-sodium
   vegetable broth

2 tablespoons tomato paste

2 tablespoons paprika

1 cup heavy (whipping) cream

½ cup sour cream

Sea salt

Freshly ground black pepper

2 tablespoons chopped fresh
   parsley, for garnish

1. Heat the olive oil in a large stockpot over medium-high heat.

2. Sauté the onion, mushrooms, and garlic until lightly caramelized, about 10 minutes.

3. Stir the tofu, vegetable broth, tomato paste, and paprika into the pot.

4. Bring the mixture to a boil, and then reduce the heat to low and simmer until the vegetables are very tender, about 10 minutes.

5. Stir in the heavy cream and sour cream.

6. Season with salt and pepper and serve topped with the parsley.

ADDITION TIP: Serve this meal over, about 4 cups chopped cauliflower sautéed in 1 tablespoon olive oil. This increases the calories to 550 and changes the macros to Fat: 80% / Carbs: 10% / Protein: 10%.

PER SERVING: Calories: 496; Total Fat: 44g; Total Carbohydrates: 12g; Net Carbs 7g; Fiber: 5g; Protein: 13g
MACROS: Fat: 80% / Carbs: 8% /Protein: 12%

Spaghetti Squash Egg Bake

SERVES 4 / PREP TIME: 15 MINUTES / COOK TIME: 1 HOUR, 10 MINUTES

500 CALORIES OR FEWER, NUT-FREE, VEGETARIAN

If you've never had spaghetti squash before, you're in for a treat. It's just like "real" pasta, folks. Spaghetti squash is a fabulous source of beta-carotene, potassium, calcium, and vitamins A, B, and C. The squash pairs nicely with the egg-and-cream base baked in this casserole.

2 tablespoons extra-virgin olive oil, plus extra for greasing the casserole dish

1 spaghetti squash, halved lengthwise and seeded

1 cup water

½ onion, chopped

1 teaspoon minced garlic

6 large eggs

2 ounces cream cheese

1 tablespoon chopped fresh basil

Sea salt

Freshly ground black pepper

1 cup grated Parmesan cheese

1. Preheat the oven to 375°F and lightly grease a 9-by-13-inch casserole dish with olive oil and set aside.
2. Place the squash cut-side down in a baking dish that fits your microwave and add 1 cup of water.
3. Microwave on high until a knife inserts easily into the flesh, 15 to 20 minutes.
4. Let the squash cool for 10 minutes, and then shred the flesh with a fork into a large bowl. Set aside.
5. While the squash is cooling, heat the oil in a medium skillet over medium-high heat and sauté the onion and garlic until softened, about 3 minutes.
6. Add the onion to the squash in the bowl along with the eggs, cream cheese, and basil and mix until well combined. Season the mixture with salt and pepper.
7. Spoon the mixture into the casserole dish and top evenly with the Parmesan cheese.
8. Cover the casserole loosely with aluminum foil and bake for 25 minutes; then remove the foil and bake until the eggs are cooked through and the top is golden, about 15 minutes more.
9. Let the casserole stand for 10 minutes before serving.

CONTINUED ▶

Spaghetti Squash Egg Bake CONTINUED

ADDITION TIP: Serve this brightly colored casserole with Blue Cheese Bok Choy Salad with Turkey (page 76). This increases the calories to 617 per serving, and the macros change to Fat: 71% / Carbs: 10% / Protein: 19%. Just remove the turkey for a vegetarian-friendly option.

PER SERVING: Calories: 363; Total Fat: 27g; Total Carbohydrates: 11g; Net Carbs: 9g; Fiber: 2g; Protein: 19g
MACROS: Fat: 67% / Carbs: 13% / Protein: 20%

Egg Cauliflower Tikka Masala

SERVES 4 / PREP TIME: 15 MINUTES / COOK TIME: 35 MINUTES

1 PAN/1 POT, NUT-FREE, VEGETARIAN

Tikka masala is a not-too-spicy curry dish with a creamy tomato-based sauce. Curry is a spice mixture—not a single spice—so not all curries taste the same. Traditional curry spices include cinnamon, cloves, coriander, cumin, ginger, paprika, and turmeric. You can also add a dash of garam masala for an authentic taste.

2 tablespoons extra-virgin olive oil

1 onion, chopped

2 teaspoons minced garlic

1 teaspoon peeled grated fresh ginger

1 head cauliflower, cut into small florets

3 tablespoons red curry paste

1 cup low-sodium vegetable broth

8 large hardboiled eggs, peeled and halved lengthwise

1 cup fresh baby spinach

2 cups heavy (whipping) cream

2 tablespoons chopped fresh cilantro, for garnish

1. Heat the olive oil in a large skillet over medium-high heat.
2. Sauté the onion, garlic, and ginger until softened, about 4 minutes.
3. Add the cauliflower and curry paste and stir to coat.
4. Add the vegetable broth and bring to a boil. Reduce the heat to low and simmer, partially covered, until the vegetables are tender, about 20 minutes.
5. Add the eggs and spinach and simmer to heat through, about 6 minutes.
6. Stir in the heavy cream and simmer for 2 minutes.
7. Serve topped with the cilantro.

VARIATION TIP: To increase the protein, whisk 2 scoops of a low-carb unflavored or vanilla protein powder into the cream before adding to the curry. This increases calories to 718 and changes the macros to Fat: 75% / Carbs: 6% / Protein: 19%.

PER SERVING: Calories: 668; Total Fat: 60g; Total Carbohydrates: 14g; Net Carbs: 11g; Fiber: 3g; Protein: 18g
MACROS: Fat: 80% / Carbs: 8% / Protein: 12%

Kale and Chard Shakshuka

SERVES 4 / PREP TIME: 15 MINUTES / COOK TIME: 20 MINUTES

1 PAN/1 POT, 500 CALORIES OR FEWER, NUT-FREE, VEGETARIAN

Shakshuka is a classic Middle Eastern breakfast dish. It's made of inexpensive ingredients such as tomatoes, eggs, greens, herbs, and cheeses. Tomatoes are the base of most shakshukas, including this recipe. Tomatoes contain lycopene, a potent antioxidant that may support heart health. And get this: When you cook tomatoes, you actually increase the lycopene content!

¼ cup extra-virgin olive oil
½ onion, diced
1 tablespoon minced garlic
4 cups chopped kale
4 cups chopped Swiss chard
½ cup chopped fresh parsley
1 (15-ounce) can low-sodium
 diced tomatoes
Juice from 1 lemon
1 teaspoon ground cumin
½ teaspoon red pepper flakes
8 large eggs
1 cup shredded
 Parmesan cheese

1. Heat the olive oil in a large skillet over medium-high heat.
2. Sauté the onion and garlic until softened, about 3 minutes.
3. Stir in the kale, Swiss chard, and parsley and sauté until the greens are wilted, about 8 minutes.
4. Stir in the tomatoes, lemon juice, cumin, and red pepper flakes and bring the mixture to a simmer.
5. Use the back of a spoon to make 8 wells in the tomato mixture, and then crack an egg into each well. Cover the skillet with a lid and let cook until the egg whites are no longer translucent, 4 to 5 minutes.
6. Remove from the heat and serve topped with the Parmesan cheese.

MAKE AHEAD: This recipe can be prepared as individual portions in 6-ounce ramekins. Make the recipe up to step 4 and evenly divide the tomato mixture among 4 ramekins. Then crack the eggs on top. Cover each ramekin and store in the refrigerator for up to 2 days. Bake from the refrigerator in a 375°F oven for about 30 minutes or until the eggs are cooked through and the base is hot.

PER SERVING: Calories: 407; Total Fat: 30g; Total Carbohydrates: 13g; Net Carbs: 9g; Fiber: 4g; Protein: 24g
MACROS: Fat: 65% / Carbs: 12% / Protein: 23%

Cheese Chili Custard

SERVES 4 / PREP TIME: 15 MINUTES / COOK TIME: 35 MINUTES

5-INGREDIENT, NUT-FREE, VEGETARIAN

Custard isn't just for dessert; it's also an elegant main course. Pair it with a mixed green salad topped with Everyday Balsamic Dressing (page 158) or Blue Cheese Dressing (page 160) and you'll be loving life. The trick to the perfect custard is the water bath, which infuses moisture by enclosing the custard in gentle heat. Make sure you use very hot water in the water bath, or it won't be effective.

2 cups coconut milk

1 cup shredded Swiss cheese

3 large eggs

3 large egg yolks

½ teaspoon chili powder

Pinch sea salt

Pinch freshly ground black pepper

1 tablespoon chopped fresh cilantro, for garnish

1. Preheat the oven to 350°F.
2. Heat the coconut milk in a medium saucepan over medium-high heat until it is just boiling, about 4 minutes; then remove from the heat and whisk in the Swiss cheese until melted.
3. In a medium bowl, beat together the eggs, yolks, chili powder, salt, and pepper.
4. Whisk the coconut milk mixture into the egg mixture until well blended.
5. Pour the egg mixture into an 8-inch round baking dish.
6. Place the baking dish in a larger square baking dish and pour boiling or very hot water into the larger baking dish so that the water level is about halfway up the side of the round dish.
7. Bake the custard until the center appears set, 25 to 30 minutes.
8. Remove the baked custard from the water bath and allow it to cool until just above room temperature.
9. Serve topped with the cilantro.

CRAVING TIP: Custard is good any time of the day, and the heat from the chili powder can curb hankerings for salty or savory foods. Also, the protein and fat from the eggs are great for controlling hunger.

PER SERVING: Calories: 512; Total Fat: 43g; Total Carbohydrates: 9g; Net Carbs: 6g; Fiber: 3g; Protein: 20g
MACROS: Fat: 76% / Carbs: 7% / Protein: 17%

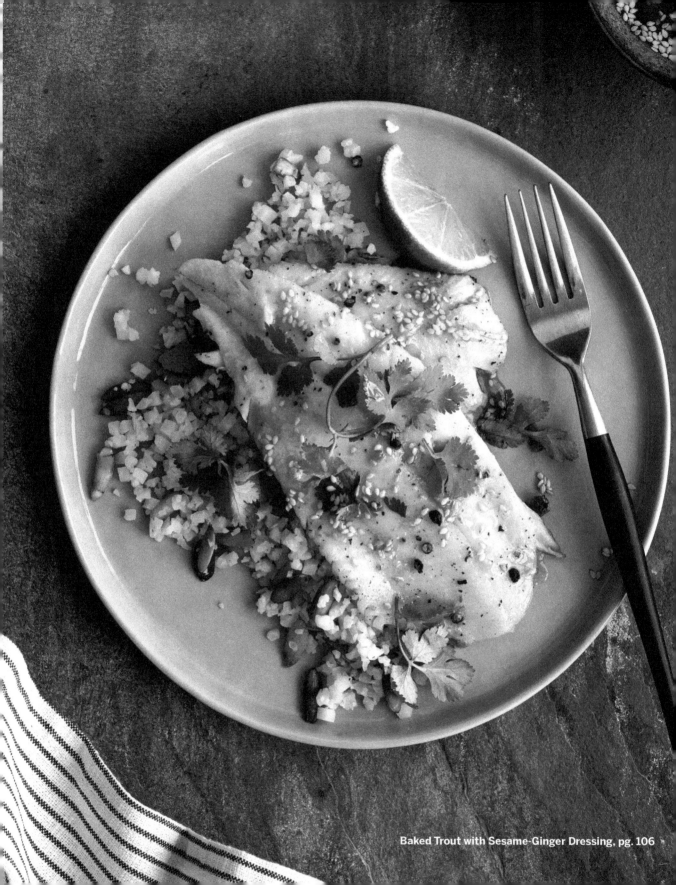

Baked Trout with Sesame-Ginger Dressing, pg. 106

CHAPTER SEVEN

Seafood & Poultry Mains

Brown Butter Baked Salmon

SERVES 4 / PREP TIME: 10 MINUTES / COOK TIME: 20 MINUTES

5-INGREDIENT, 30-MINUTE, 500 CALORIES OR FEWER, NUT-FREE

This simple meal highlights the distinct flavor and texture of salmon, a staple keto protein. When you pair this fish with brown butter—a caramelized, toffee-like creation—you make culinary magic. If possible, look for wild-caught Pacific salmon from the Canadian or U.S. coast. These fish have high levels of omega-3 fatty acids and vitamin D.

1 tablespoon extra-virgin olive oil, plus more for greasing the baking sheet
4 (4-ounce) salmon fillets
Sea salt
Freshly ground black pepper
⅓ cup butter
1 teaspoon chopped fresh thyme, for garnish

1. Preheat the oven to 350°F. Line a baking sheet with aluminum foil and lightly grease it with olive oil.
2. Pat the salmon fillets dry with paper towels, season with salt and pepper, and place on the prepared baking sheet.
3. Drizzle the fish with 1 tablespoon of olive oil and bake until the fish is cooked through, 18 to 20 minutes.
4. While the fish is baking, place the butter in a small skillet over medium heat.
5. Melt the butter, whisking constantly and swirling the melted butter until brown flecks appear at the bottom of the skillet.
6. Remove the skillet from the heat and continue whisking until the butter is very fragrant and light brown.
7. Drizzle the cooked fish with the brown butter and serve topped with the thyme.

ADDITION TIP: Serve this dish alongside a portion of Sesame Tofu Broccoli Fried Rice (page 95) for a 690-calorie meal. The macros for this pairing would be Fat: 70% / Carbs: 7% / Protein: 23%

PER SERVING: Calories: 362; Total Fat: 30g; Total Carbohydrates: 0g; Net Carbs: 0g; Fiber: 0g; Protein: 23g
MACROS: Fat: 75% / Carbs: 0% / Protein: 25%

Baked Nutty Halibut

SERVES 4 / PREP TIME: 20 MINUTES / COOK TIME: 15 MINUTES

5-INGREDIENT, 500 CALORIES OR FEWER

Nuts and fish are a natural culinary alliance because the oil-packed nuts keep the fish moist while it bakes. The almonds in this dish have a subtle buttery flavor that isn't obscured by the pecan topping. Almonds are packed with monounsaturated fats and beneficial fiber, both of which support a healthy heart.

½ cup heavy (whipping) cream
½ cup finely chopped pecans
¼ cup finely chopped almonds
4 (4-ounce) boneless halibut fillets
Sea salt
Freshly ground black pepper
2 tablespoons extra-virgin olive oil

1. Preheat the oven to 400°F. Line a baking sheet with parchment.
2. Pour the heavy cream into a bowl and set it on your work surface.
3. In another bowl, stir together the pecans and almonds and set beside the cream.
4. Pat the halibut fillets dry with paper towels and lightly season with salt and pepper.
5. Dip the fillets in the cream, shaking off the excess; then dredge the fish in the nut mixture so that both sides of each piece are thickly coated.
6. Place the fish on the prepared baking sheet and brush both sides of the pieces generously with olive oil.
7. Bake the fish until the topping is golden and the fish flakes easily with a fork, 12 to 15 minutes. Serve.

MAKE AHEAD: The "breaded" fish fillets can be completely put together and then frozen on a baking sheet. Transfer the individual fillets to plastic bags and freeze for up to 1 month. Cook the fillets from frozen, brushed lightly with olive oil, in a 350°F oven for about 35 minutes.

PER SERVING: Calories: 392; Total Fat: 31g; Total Carbohydrates: 3g; Net Carbs: 1g; Fiber: 2g; Protein: 26g
MACROS: Fat: 70% / Carbs: 3% / Protein: 27%

Baked Trout with Sesame-Ginger Dressing

SERVES 4 / PREP TIME: 10 MINUTES / COOK TIME: 15 MINUTES

1 PAN/1 POT, 5-INGREDIENT, 30-MINUTE, 500 CALORIES OR FEWER, DAIRY-FREE, NUT-FREE

Trout is high in protein, omega-3 fatty acids, potassium, and B vitamins, which makes it a great choice for a healthy diet. Rainbow trout, you'll want to know, is one of the least contaminated farmed fish.

4 (3-ounce) trout fillets
Sea salt
Freshly ground black pepper
½ cup Sesame-Ginger Dressing (page 159)
1 tablespoon chopped fresh cilantro, for garnish
1 lime, quartered, for garnish

1. Preheat the oven to 400°F.
2. Pat the trout fillets dry with paper towels; then lightly season with salt and pepper and place in a single layer in a 9-by-9-inch baking dish.
3. Spoon 1 tablespoon of dressing on each piece of fish.
4. Bake until the fish is just cooked through, 12 to 14 minutes.
5. Spoon the remaining dressing over the fish and serve topped with the cilantro and lime wedges.

ADDITION TIP: Pair this dish with Cauliflower Pumpkin Seed Couscous (page 87) or Fiery Coconut Noodles (page 90) for a more filling meal. This increases the calories to 803 or 673, respectively.

PER SERVING: Calories: 297; Total Fat: 24g; Total Carbohydrates: 1g; Net Carbs: 1g; Fiber: 0g; Protein: 20g
MACROS: Fat: 72% / Carbs: 2% / Protein: 26%

Cream-Poached Trout

SERVES 4 / PREP TIME: 10 MINUTES / COOK TIME: 20 MINUTES

30-MINUTE, 500 CALORIES OR FEWER, NUT-FREE

If you've never had poached fish with cream, you're in for a treat. The leeks pair well with the sweetness of the cream in this dish but don't overpower the flavors as an onion might. Leeks contain kaempferol, a flavonoid that researchers believe may benefit the heart. Take the time to clean your leeks after slicing them because they are often filled with grit.

4 (4-ounce) skinless
  trout fillets
Sea salt
Freshly ground black pepper
3 tablespoons butter
1 leek, white and green parts,
  halved lengthwise, thinly
  sliced, and
  thoroughly washed
1 teaspoon minced garlic
1 cup heavy (whipping) cream
Juice of 1 lemon
1 teaspoon chopped fresh
  parsley, for garnish

1. Preheat the oven to 400°F.
2. Pat the trout fillets dry with paper towels and lightly season with salt and pepper. Place them in a 9-by-9-inch baking dish in one layer. Set aside.
3. Place a medium saucepan over medium-high heat and melt the butter.
4. Sauté the leek and garlic until softened, about 6 minutes.
5. Add the heavy cream and lemon juice to the saucepan and bring to a boil, whisking.
6. Pour the sauce over the fish and bake until the fish is just cooked through, 10 to 12 minutes.
7. Serve topped with the parsley.

ADDITION TIP: Serve the trout with Cauliflower Pumpkin Seed Couscous (page 87) for a balanced meal of 973 calories, 77 grams of fat, and 50 grams of protein. The macros would be Fat: 71% / Carbs: 8% / Protein: 21%.

PER SERVING: Calories: 449; Total Fat: 37g; Total Carbohydrates: 5g; Net Carbs: 4g; Fiber: 1g; Protein: 24g
MACROS: Fat: 74% / Carbs: 5% / Protein: 21%

Fish Avocado Tacos

SERVES 4 / PREP TIME: 20 MINUTES / COOKING TIME: 15 MINUTES

500 CALORIES OR FEWER, NUT-FREE

Fish tacos are hot these days. Why? Because they're delicious! Cumin is the most prominent flavor in this recipe, and its peppery flavor pairs well with the salmon. Cumin is high in iron and also contains calcium, manganese, and magnesium—key minerals for supporting bone health.

4 (4-ounce) salmon fillets
1 teaspoon ground cumin
⅛ teaspoon cayenne pepper
Sea salt
2 tablespoons extra-virgin olive oil
½ cup avocado oil mayonnaise
¼ cup sour cream
1 teaspoon sriracha sauce
Juice of 1 lime
1 cup shredded cabbage
1 carrot, shredded
1 cup shredded celery root
4 large lettuce leaves
1 avocado, diced
1 tablespoon finely chopped fresh cilantro

1. Preheat the oven to 350°F.
2. Pat the salmon fillets dry with paper towels and place them in a single layer in a 9-by-9-inch baking dish.
3. Season the fish lightly with the cumin, cayenne, and salt.
4. Drizzle the fish with the olive oil and bake until just cooked through, 12 to 15 minutes.
5. While the fish is baking, stir together the mayonnaise, sour cream, sriracha sauce, and lime juice in a medium bowl until well blended.
6. Stir in the cabbage, carrot, and celery root until mixed.
7. When the fish is cooked, arrange the lettuce leaves on your work surface and place a fish fillet in the center of each.
8. Top with the slaw, avocado, and cilantro and serve.

MAKE AHEAD: The slaw topping can be made 2 to 3 days ahead and stored sealed in the refrigerator. Break it out and use it as a topping for pork, poultry, or other meals.

PER SERVING: Calories: 498; Total Fat: 40g; Total Carbohydrates: 11g; Net Carbs: 6g; Fiber: 5g; Protein: 25g
MACROS: Fat: 71% / Carbs: 9% / Protein: 20%

Fish Coconut Curry

SERVES 4 / PREP TIME: 15 MINUTES / COOK TIME: 30 MINUTES

1 PAN/1 POT, NUT-FREE

The quality of a fish stew depends, in large part, on the type of fish used. The calorie, fat, and protein levels will vary in this recipe as you mix up your fish choices. Salmon was used in the calculations here. If you use a different fish, you will have to adjust the macros and calories on your fast day.

¼ cup coconut oil

1 onion, chopped

1 tablespoon minced garlic

1 tablespoon minced jalapeño pepper

1 tablespoon peeled grated fresh ginger

1 cup diced eggplant

2 zucchini, diced

1½ tablespoons curry powder

½ teaspoon ground cumin

1 cup heavy (whipping) cream

1 cup low-sodium chicken broth

2 cups green beans, cut into 1-inch pieces

1 pound firm fish, cut into 1-inch chunks

1 cup fresh baby spinach

1. Heat the coconut oil in a large saucepan over medium-high heat.
2. Sauté the onion, garlic, jalapeño, and ginger until softened, about 5 minutes.
3. Add the eggplant and zucchini and sauté for 5 minutes.
4. Stir in the curry powder and cumin and sauté until very fragrant, about 2 minutes.
5. Stir in the heavy cream and chicken broth and bring the liquid to a boil.
6. Reduce the heat to low and simmer until the vegetables are tender, about 5 minutes.
7. Stir in the green beans and fish and simmer until the fish is cooked through, 8 to 10 minutes.
8. Stir in the spinach and let the curry stand for 5 minutes off the heat to wilt the spinach. Serve.

SUBSTITUTION TIP: For a vegetarian dish, use pressed and diced tofu instead of fish in the same amount. Sauté the tofu in coconut oil until crispy (in step 2) and remove it to a plate. Add the tofu back in step 7 and follow the directions as written.

PER SERVING: Calories: 505; Total Fat: 39g; Total Carbohydrates: 15g; Net Carbs: 9g; Fiber: 6g; Protein: 24g
MACROS: Fat: 70% / Carbs: 10% / Protein: 20%

Chili Seafood Stew

SERVES 6 / PREP TIME: 15 MINUTES / COOK TIME: 35 MINUTES

1 PAN/1 POT, 500 CALORIES OR FEWER, DAIRY-FREE, NUT-FREE

This stew has many layers of flavor: sweet potato, celery, coconut, red pepper flakes, and the mild licorice taste of fresh fennel. Fennel is an elegant-looking vegetable with a curved shape that looks a little like a musical instrument. A member of the carrot family, fennel is an excellent source of vitamin C, potassium, fiber, and folate. It's topped with feathery fronds, which make a perfect garnish.

¼ cup coconut oil

1 onion, chopped

2 celery stalks, chopped

1 tablespoon minced garlic

½ fennel bulb, thinly sliced

1 sweet potato, diced

1 carrot, diced

1 (15-ounce) can low-sodium diced tomatoes

1 cup low-sodium chicken broth

1 cup coconut milk

¼ teaspoon red pepper flakes

12 ounces firm fish, cut into 1-inch chunks (salmon, halibut, haddock)

2 tablespoons chopped fresh cilantro, for garnish

1. Heat the coconut oil in a large stockpot over medium-high heat.

2. Sauté the onion, celery, and garlic until softened, about 4 minutes.

3. Add the fennel, sweet potato, and carrot and sauté for 4 minutes more.

4. Stir in the tomatoes, broth, coconut milk, and red pepper flakes and bring the stew to a boil.

5. Reduce the heat to low and simmer until the vegetables are tender, about 15 minutes.

6. Stir in the fish and simmer until it is cooked through, about 10 minutes.

7. Serve topped with the cilantro.

ADDITION TIP: Add 8 ounces of chopped pancetta or bacon in step 2 for flavor, fat, and protein. This addition increases the calories to 446 per serving and the macros to Fat: 77% / Carbs: 6% / Protein: 17%.

PER SERVING: Calories: 277; Total Fat: 21g; Total Carbohydrates: 7g; Net Carbs: 4g; Fiber: 3g; Protein: 14g
MACROS: Fat: 70% / Carbs: 10% / Protein: 20%

Shrimp and Sausage Sauté

SERVES 4 / PREP TIME: 15 MINUTES / COOK TIME: 20 MINUTES

500 CALORIES OR FEWER, DAIRY-FREE, NUT-FREE

If you like fajitas, this dish will please your palate. Shrimp, sausage, and bell peppers all combine in one skillet toss. All colors of bell pepper contain vitamins A (beta-carotene), B, C, and E as well as calcium, magnesium, and zinc. These nutrients are crucial for immunity, energy, skin health, bone health, and much more.

3 tablespoons extra-virgin olive oil, divided

8 ounces (31–35 count) raw shrimp, peeled, deveined, and tails removed

8 ounces cooked hot Italian sausage, diced

2 green bell peppers, cut into strips

1 red bell pepper, cut into strips

½ onion, thinly sliced

2 teaspoons minced garlic

1 teaspoon chopped fresh oregano

1 teaspoon ground cumin

1. Heat 2 tablespoons of olive oil in a large skillet over medium-high heat.

2. Sauté the shrimp until it is just cooked through, about 5 minutes. With a slotted spoon, remove the shrimp to a plate and cover with aluminum foil to keep warm. Set aside.

3. Add the remaining 1 tablespoon of oil to the skillet and sauté the sausage, bell peppers, onion, garlic, oregano, and cumin until the sausage is heated through and the vegetables are tender and lightly browned, 10 to 12 minutes.

4. Return the shrimp to the skillet and sauté for 5 minutes more. Serve.

SUBSTITUTION TIP: If you need to avoid seafood, use diced chicken thigh or breast as your protein. Increase the cooking time for the poultry in step 2 by 5 minutes. This will ensure that it's cooked through.

PER SERVING: Calories: 281; Total Fat: 21g; Total Carbohydrates: 7g; Net Carbs: 5g; Fiber: 2g; Protein: 16g
MACROS: Fat: 67% / Carbs: 10% / Protein: 23%

Turkey Sausage Meatloaf

SERVES 6 / PREP TIME: 10 MINUTES / COOK TIME: 1 HOUR, 15 MINUTES

500 CALORIES OR FEWER

Meatloaf is a two-meal creation; it's just as good the next day. The shredded carrot ensures a moist loaf and adds a dash of color to the dish. Carrots are high in beta-carotene, a nutrient that supports eye health and immunity.

2 tablespoons extra-virgin olive oil

½ onion, chopped

1 carrot, shredded

2 teaspoons minced garlic

1 pound ground turkey

8 ounces turkey sausage meat

½ cup heavy (whipping) cream

1 large egg

½ cup ground almonds

1 tablespoon chopped fresh parsley

Pinch sea salt

Pinch freshly ground black pepper

1. Preheat the oven to 350°F.
2. Heat the olive oil in a small skillet over medium-high heat.
3. Sauté the onion, carrot, and garlic until softened, about 5 minutes.
4. Transfer the vegetables to a large bowl and add the ground turkey, sausage, heavy cream, egg, ground almonds, parsley, salt, and pepper.
5. Mix until the ingredients hold together, and then press the mixture into a 9-by-5-inch loaf pan.
6. Bake until cooked through and golden, 60 to 70 minutes.
7. Let the meatloaf rest for 10 minutes before serving.

MAKE AHEAD: Meatloaf is a classic make-and-freeze meal. Cook the meatloaf, cool, and freeze in individual portions sealed in freezer-friendly plastic bags for up to 3 months. You can also double the portion to create 710-calorie choices.

PER SERVING: Calories: 355; Total Fat: 28g; Total Carbohydrates: 6g; Net Carbs: 3g; Fiber: 3g; Protein: 21g
MACROS: Fat: 70% / Carbs: 6% / Protein: 24%

Frittata with Turkey and Spinach

SERVES 4 / PREP TIME: 15 MINUTES / COOK TIME: 30 MINUTES

500 CALORIES OR FEWER, NUT-FREE

Zucchini adds nutrients without a strong flavor. Plus the color adds a pleasing contrast to this egg-based dish. Green and yellow zucchini work equally well. If you don't enjoy large seeds, avoid the yellow variety.

6 large eggs

½ cup heavy (whipping) cream

Sea salt

Freshly ground black pepper

3 tablespoons extra-virgin olive oil

½ onion, chopped

2 teaspoons minced garlic

2 cups fresh baby spinach

2 yellow zucchini, shredded

8 ounces cooked turkey breast, diced

1. Preheat the oven to 375°F.
2. In a small bowl, whisk together the eggs and heavy cream. Season with salt and pepper and set aside.
3. Heat the olive oil in a large oven-safe skillet over medium-high heat.
4. Sauté the onion and garlic until softened, about 3 minutes.
5. Add the spinach and zucchini and cook until the spinach is wilted, about 4 minutes.
6. Add the turkey and stir to combine.
7. Pour the egg mixture into the skillet and cook until the egg sets on the bottom, about 3 minutes.
8. Bake the frittata until a knife inserted in the center comes out clean, about 20 minutes. Serve.

MAKE AHEAD: Prepare the frittata; then cool, portion, and freeze in resealable plastic bags for up to 1 month. Microwave on high for 2 minutes to reheat, and then add to salads or lettuce wraps.

PER SERVING: Calories: 433; Total Fat: 33g; Total Carbohydrates: 7g; Net Carbs: 5g; Fiber: 2g; Protein: 27g
MACROS: Fat: 70% / Carbs: 6% / Protein: 24%

Chicken Thighs in Buttery Lemon Sauce

SERVES 4 / PREP TIME: 10 MINUTES / COOK TIME: 35 MINUTES

500 CALORIES OR FEWER, NUT-FREE

Chicken thighs are juicier and less costly than their blander counterpart: chicken breasts. The creamy sauce in this dish includes butter, cream, lemon juice, chicken broth, and garlic. It's simple yet delicious.

4 (4-ounce) boneless, skinless chicken thighs
Sea salt
Freshly ground black pepper
1 tablespoon extra-virgin olive oil
3 tablespoons butter
1 tablespoon minced garlic
½ cup heavy (whipping) cream
½ cup low-sodium chicken broth
Juice of ½ lemon
1 tablespoon chopped fresh basil, for garnish

1. Preheat the oven to 400°F.
2. Pat the chicken dry with paper towels and lightly season with salt and pepper.
3. Heat the olive oil in a large oven-safe skillet over medium-high heat.
4. Pan sear the chicken until golden brown, about 4 minutes. Turn the chicken and cook the other side, about 4 minutes. Remove the thighs to a plate and set aside.
5. Add the butter to the skillet and sauté the garlic until softened, about 2 minutes.
6. Whisk in the heavy cream, chicken broth, and lemon juice.
7. Bring the sauce to a boil, and then return the chicken to the skillet.
8. Cover the skillet with a lid or with aluminum foil and braise the chicken in the oven until it is cooked through, 20 to 25 minutes.
9. Serve topped with the basil.

VARIATION TIP: The creamy sauce in this recipe also pairs well with fish such as trout or halibut. If you go the fish route, reduce the cook time to 20 minutes.

PER SERVING: Calories: 379; Total Fat: 31g; Total Carbohydrates: 2g; Net Carbs: 2g; Fiber: 0g; Protein: 23g
MACROS: Fat: 74% / Carbs: 2% / Protein: 24%

Chicken Chow Mein

SERVES 4 / PREP TIME: 20 MINUTES / COOK TIME: 25 MINUTES

500 CALORIES OR FEWER, DAIRY-FREE

This chow mein is missing the base noodles but is nonetheless close to the classic dish. If you want to add noodles, toss in konjac noodles along with the sauce. This extra ingredient doesn't change the macros much, only adding about 25 calories per portion.

FOR THE SAUCE

- ½ cup low-sodium chicken broth
- 2 tablespoons coconut aminos
- 2 tablespoons rice vinegar
- 1 tablespoon fish sauce
- 1 tablespoon granulated erythritol
- 1 tablespoon coconut oil
- 1 tablespoon almond flour

FOR THE CHOW MEIN

- 3 tablespoons extra-virgin olive oil
- 12 ounces boneless, skinless chicken breast, diced
- 1 tablespoon sesame oil
- 1 teaspoon minced garlic
- 2 cups shredded Napa cabbage
- 2 cups bean sprouts
- 1 carrot, shredded
- 1 cup snow peas, stringed and julienned
- 2 scallions, green parts only, chopped

TO MAKE THE SAUCE

In a small bowl, stir together the chicken broth, coconut aminos, rice vinegar, fish sauce, erythritol, coconut oil, and almond flour until well blended. Set aside.

TO MAKE THE CHOW MEIN

1. Heat the olive oil in a large skillet over medium-high heat.
2. Sauté the chicken until just cooked through, about 8 minutes. With a slotted spoon, remove the chicken to a plate and set aside.
3. Add the sesame oil to the skillet and sauté the garlic until softened, about 2 minutes.
4. Stir in the cabbage, bean sprouts, and carrot and sauté until tender-crisp, about 6 minutes.
5. Stir in the snow peas and scallions and sauté for 4 minutes.
6. Move the vegetables to one side of the skillet; then pour the sauce in the other side and cook until it thickens, about 2 minutes.
7. Return the chicken to the skillet and toss everything together. Serve.

SUBSTITUTION TIP: For a vegan/vegetarian meal, omit the chicken and add 1 pound of extra-firm tofu. Prepare the tofu the same as the chicken, including the cooking time. This changes the macros to Fat: 72% / Carbs: 14% / Protein: 14%.

PER SERVING: Calories: 406; Total Fat: 30g; Total Carbohydrates: 13g; Net Carbs: 9g; Fiber: 4g; Protein: 21g; Erythritol Carbs: 3g
MACROS: Fat: 67% / Carbs: 12% / Protein: 21%

Golden Chicken Asiago

SERVES 4 / PREP TIME: 15 MINUTES / COOK TIME: 15 MINUTES

30-MINUTE

This recipe is similar to a classic chicken Parmesan, but with Asiago instead. Use the cutlets as a main course or chop them up and put them on your salad. To avoid a mess when making this dish, use one hand for wet (dipping) while the other stays dry.

2 large eggs
2 tablespoons heavy (whipping) cream
1 cup almond flour, divided
1 cup grated Asiago cheese
4 (4-ounce) boneless, skinless chicken breasts, pounded to a ½-inch thickness
¼ cup extra-virgin olive oil
½ cup mayonnaise
1 tablespoon hot sauce

1. In a small bowl, whisk the eggs and heavy cream together and set aside.
2. Place ½ cup of almond flour in another bowl and set beside the egg mixture.
3. In a third bowl, stir together the remaining ½ cup of almond flour and the Asiago cheese.
4. Dredge one piece of chicken in the almond flour, then in the egg mixture, and then the cheese mixture. Repeat with the remaining chicken.
5. Heat the olive oil in a large skillet over medium-high heat and panfry the chicken until cooked through and browned on both sides, turning once, about 15 minutes in total.
6. In a small bowl, stir together the mayonnaise and hot sauce.
7. Serve the chicken with the sauce.

MAKE AHEAD: Feel free to freeze and store these cutlets, cooked or uncooked. Cooked chicken can be thawed in the refrigerator overnight or reheated in the oven or microwave. Uncooked chicken cutlets can be baked straight from frozen in a 350°F oven for 30 minutes.

PER SERVING: Calories: 532; Total Fat: 39g; Total Carbohydrates: 8g; Net Carbs: 6g; Fiber: 2g; Protein: 36g
MACROS: Fat: 65% / Carbs: 6% / Protein: 29%

Pecan-Stuffed Chicken Thighs

SERVES 4 / PREP TIME: 20 MINUTES / COOK TIME: 25 MINUTES

5-INGREDIENT

If you need a fancy dish to serve guests, look no further than these nut-and-cheese-stuffed thighs. Guests will love the sun-dried tomatoes, which add both salty flavor and visual nuance to the presentation. For optimal taste, look for sun-dried tomatoes packed in seasoned olive oil. (Just pat the excess oil off with a paper towel.) A little bit of sun-dried tomatoes goes a long way.

4 ounces goat cheese

½ cup chopped pecans

2 tablespoons chopped sun-dried tomatoes

4 (5-ounce) skin-on, boneless chicken thighs, butterflied

Sea salt

Freshly ground black pepper

2 tablespoons extra-virgin olive oil

¼ cup low-sodium chicken broth

1. Preheat the oven to 350°F.
2. In a small bowl, stir together the goat cheese, pecans, and sun-dried tomatoes until well mixed.
3. Pat the chicken thighs dry with a paper towel. Use your fingers to loosen the skin on one thigh so that it forms a pocket still connected at the edges.
4. Carefully spoon the goat cheese mixture into the pocket and pull the skin back to cover the filling. Repeat with the remaining chicken.
5. Season the chicken with salt and pepper.
6. Heat the olive oil in a large oven-safe skillet over medium-high heat.
7. Pan sear the chicken, skin-side down, until the skin is crispy and golden, about 5 minutes.
8. Turn the chicken over and add the chicken broth to the skillet. Cover with a lid or aluminum foil and bake until the chicken is cooked through to about 165°F internal temperature, about 20 minutes. Serve.

VARIATION TIP: If you prefer, stuff the filling into butterflied pork chops instead of chicken. Just secure the edges of the chops with toothpicks to ensure that the filling doesn't ooze out.

PER SERVING: Calories: 554; Total Fat: 48g; Total Carbohydrates: 3g; Net Carbs: 1g; Fiber: 2g; Protein: 28g
MACROS: Fat: 77% / Carbs: 3% / Protein: 20%

Chicken Tenders with Creamy Almond Sauce

SERVES 4 / PREP TIME: 12 MINUTES / COOK TIME: 20 MINUTES

30-MINUTE

You can use either chicken breasts or chicken tenders (which are less expensive) for this recipe. To mix things up, serve the tenders without creamy almond sauce as a lettuce wrap base or in a salad. These tenders can be prepared and frozen (raw or cooked) for up to three months.

FOR THE ALMOND SAUCE
½ cup heavy (whipping) cream
2 tablespoons almond butter
Juice of 1 lime
1 teaspoon coconut aminos

FOR THE CHICKEN TENDERS
2 large eggs, beaten
1½ cups almond flour
12 ounces boneless chicken, cut into ½-inch wide strips
3 tablespoons extra-virgin olive oil

TO MAKE THE ALMOND SAUCE

In a small bowl, whisk together the heavy cream, almond butter, lime juice, and coconut aminos until well blended. Set aside.

TO MAKE THE CHICKEN TENDERS

1. Preheat the oven to 400°F. Line a baking sheet with parchment paper and set aside.
2. Place the small bowl of beaten eggs on your work surface.
3. Place the almond flour in another small bowl and set it beside the egg mixture.
4. Dredge the chicken in the almond flour, then the egg mixture, and then back in the almond flour.
5. Place the breaded tenders on the prepared baking sheet and brush all sides with the olive oil.
6. Bake until the chicken is cooked through and golden, turning once, 15 to 18 minutes in total.
7. Serve with the almond sauce.

SUBSTITUTION OR VARIATION TIP: If you have a tree nut allergy, omit the sauce altogether and use shredded unsweetened coconut instead of ground almond for your "breading." This changes the calories to 515 and the macros to Fat: 71% / Carbs: 8% / Protein: 21%.

PER SERVING: Calories: 555; Total Fat: 46g; Total Carbohydrates: 8g; Net Carbs: 6g; Fiber: 2g; Protein: 29g
MACROS: Fat: 72% / Carbs: 6% / Protein: 22%

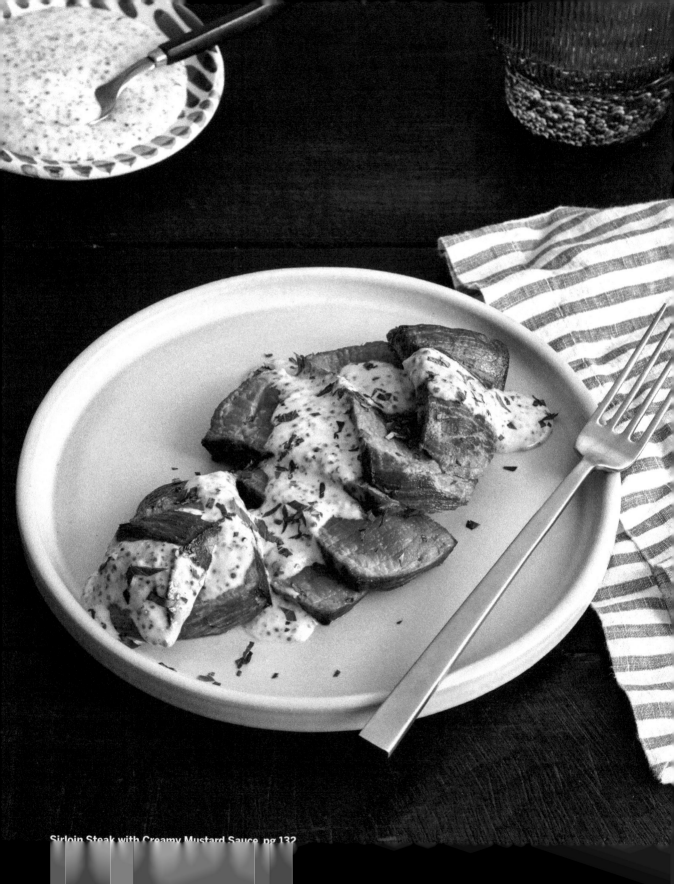

Sirloin Steak with Creamy Mustard Sauce, pg 132

CHAPTER EIGHT

Pork & Beef Mains

Pork and Mashed Cauliflower Shepherd's Pie

SERVES 8 / PREP TIME: 15 MINUTES / COOK TIME: 55 MINUTES

500 CALORIES OR FEWER, NUT-FREE

You will definitely have leftovers from this recipe. So rich, so hearty. Store leftovers in the freezer, and thaw, heat, and serve when you want a quick and satisfying meal.

½ head cauliflower, cut into florets

2 tablespoons butter

¼ cup heavy (whipping) cream

Sea salt

Freshly ground black pepper

2 tablespoons extra-virgin olive oil

1 pound ground pork

1 onion, chopped

1 tablespoon minced garlic

1 cup low-sodium diced tomatoes

1 cup frozen peas

1 teaspoon Worcestershire sauce

1 teaspoon chopped fresh oregano

1 cup shredded Cheddar cheese

1. Bring a large saucepan of water to a boil over high heat.
2. Boil the cauliflower until tender, about 10 minutes.
3. Drain the water out of the saucepan and add the butter and heavy cream to the cauliflower. Mash until smooth and creamy and season with salt and pepper. Set aside.
4. Heat the olive oil in a large skillet over medium-high heat.
5. Sauté the pork until cooked through, about 7 minutes.
6. Add the onion and garlic and sauté for 3 minutes.
7. Remove the meat mixture from the heat and stir in the tomatoes, peas, Worcestershire sauce, and oregano.
8. Spread the meat mixture in a 9-by-13-inch baking dish and spread the mashed cauliflower evenly over the meat mixture.
9. Top the casserole with the Cheddar cheese and bake until bubbly and golden brown, about 35 minutes. Serve.

ADDITION TIP: Double the portion to create a 572-calorie meal. The macros are spot-on for keto.

PER SERVING: Calories: 286; Total Fat: 22g; Total Carbohydrates: 7g; Net Carbs: 5g; Fiber: 2g; Protein: 15g
MACROS: Fat: 70% / Carbs: 9% / Protein: 21%

Jerk Pork Tenderloin

SERVES 6 / PREP TIME: 15 MINUTES / COOK TIME: 20 MINUTES

500 CALORIES OR FEWER, NUT-FREE

Pork tenderloin is a lean cut of meat, so it's not the first choice for keto. Nonetheless, it's still a nutritious protein source. Plus pork tastes so mild, it goes with nearly anything. Adding a dollop of sour cream or a mayonnaise-based topping (as in this recipe) bumps up your macros to keto-approved levels.

1 tablespoon granulated erythritol

½ tablespoon garlic powder

½ tablespoon ground allspice

½ tablespoon dried thyme

1 teaspoon ground cinnamon

¼ teaspoon salt

¼ teaspoon freshly ground black pepper

⅛ teaspoon cayenne pepper

1 (1-pound) pork tenderloin, cut into 1-inch rounds

¼ cup extra-virgin olive oil

½ cup sour cream

2 tablespoons chopped fresh cilantro, for garnish

1. In a medium bowl, stir together the erythritol, garlic powder, allspice, thyme, cinnamon, salt, pepper, and cayenne.
2. Rub the pork pieces generously on all sides with the seasoning mixture.
3. Heat the olive oil in a large skillet over medium-high heat.
4. Panfry the pork until just cooked through, turning once, about 20 minutes in total.
5. Serve topped with the sour cream and cilantro.

VARIATION TIP: Try the jerk seasoning with beef, chicken, salmon, and shrimp, too. Double or triple the seasoning and store sealed at room temperature for up to 3 months.

PER SERVING: Calories: 287; Total Fat: 23g; Total Carbohydrates: 3g; Net Carbs: 2g; Fiber: 1g; Protein: 17g; Erythritol carbs: 2g
MACROS: Fat: 72% / Carbs: 4% / Protein: 24%

Pork Pumpkin Ragout

SERVES 6 / PREP TIME: 15 MINUTES / COOK TIME: 45 MINUTES

1 PAN/1 POT, NUT-FREE

Ragout is, quite simply, a meat-and-vegetable stew slow-cooked to perfection with spices and herbs. The pumpkin in this dish adds both sweetness and nutrients. Pumpkin is a superb source of fiber, beta-carotene, iron, and vitamins B, C, and E as well as potassium, which helps maintain healthy blood pressure.

2 tablespoons extra-virgin olive oil

1 pound pork center loin chops, cut into 1½-inch chunks

2 cups cubed pumpkin (1-inch chunks)

1 red bell pepper, diced

½ onion, halved and sliced

1 tablespoon minced garlic

1½ cups low-sodium chicken broth

1½ cups coconut milk

2 teaspoons chopped fresh thyme

½ cup heavy (whipping) cream

Salt

Freshly ground black pepper

8 slices cooked bacon, chopped

1. Heat the olive oil in a large stockpot over medium-high heat and sauté the pork until it is cooked through, about 7 minutes.
2. Add the pumpkin, bell pepper, onion, and garlic and sauté until the vegetables are softened, about 10 minutes.
3. Stir in the chicken broth, coconut milk, and thyme and bring the mixture to a boil.
4. Reduce the heat to low and simmer until the vegetables and meat are tender, about 25 minutes.
5. Stir in the heavy cream and season with salt and pepper.
6. Serve topped with the bacon.

MAKE AHEAD: Make this stew in bulk. Pro tip: Leave out the heavy cream and bacon when freezing. This prevents the stew from splitting and the bacon from drooping. Add these ingredients when you reheat.

PER SERVING: Calories: 526; Total Fat: 42g; Total Carbohydrates: 10g; Net Carbs: 7g; Fiber: 3g; Protein: 27g
MACROS: Fat: 71% / Carbs: 8% / Protein: 21%

Brussels Sprout Ground Pork Hash

SERVES 4 / PREP TIME: 15 MINUTES / COOK TIME: 30 MINUTES

500 CALORIES OR FEWER, ALLERGEN-FREE

People either love or hate Brussels sprouts. Often, bad childhood experiences with this sulfurous vegetable are to blame. To avoid overcooking Brussels sprouts, do a quick sauté on the stovetop or roast them in the oven until slightly tender. Brussels sprouts are extremely high in fiber, iron, vitamins A and C, and potassium as well as a good source of vitamins B, E, and K. Special compounds in Brussels sprouts called isothiocyanates have been shown to have anticancer effects.

3 tablespoons extra-virgin olive oil, divided

8 ounces ground pork

4 bacon slices, chopped

½ onion, chopped

1 tablespoon minced garlic

8 ounces Brussels sprouts, trimmed and sliced

1 sweet potato, diced

Juice of 1 lemon

1 teaspoon chopped fresh parsley

Sea salt

Freshly ground black pepper

1. Heat 1 tablespoon of olive oil in a large skillet over medium-high heat.
2. Sauté the pork and bacon until cooked through, about 7 minutes. With a slotted spoon, remove the meat to a plate and set aside.
3. Add the remaining 2 tablespoons of olive oil to the skillet and sauté the onion and garlic until softened, about 3 minutes.
4. Stir in the Brussels sprouts and sweet potato and sauté until the vegetables are tender, 18 to 20 minutes.
5. Stir in the reserved pork and bacon, lemon juice, and parsley.
6. Season with salt and pepper and serve.

ADDITION TIP: Increase your fat intake by finishing this meal with a couple of Pumpkin Pecan Fat Bombs (page 144). This "dessert" adds 200 calories and 20 grams of healthy fat.

PER SERVING: Calories: 353; Total Fat: 26g; Total Carbohydrates: 12g; Net Carbs: 8g; Fiber: 4g; Protein: 20g
MACROS: Fat: 65% / Carbs: 12% / Protein: 23%

Spicy Pork Lettuce Wraps

SERVES 4 / PREP TIME: 15 MINUTES / COOK TIME: 20 MINUTES

500 CALORIES OR FEWER, DAIRY-FREE

Who needs tortillas and pita bread when you have fresh lettuce? Lettuce wraps are popular as a snack or an appetizer, but you can also create main course wraps with nutritious fillings. In this recipe, the spicy pork and vegetable combination contains enough calories to make a full meal.

FOR THE SAUCE

2 tablespoons coconut oil

1 tablespoon rice vinegar

1 tablespoon granulated erythritol

1 tablespoon fish sauce

1 tablespoon almond flour

1 teaspoon coconut aminos

FOR THE WRAPS

2 tablespoons sesame oil, divided

1 pound ground pork

1 teaspoon minced garlic

1 teaspoon peeled grated fresh ginger

1 red bell pepper, seeded and thinly sliced

1 carrot, peeled and grated

1 scallion, white and green parts, thinly sliced

8 large romaine or Boston lettuce leaves

TO MAKE THE SAUCE

Whisk together the coconut oil, rice vinegar, erythritol, fish sauce, almond flour, and coconut aminos in a small bowl. Set aside.

TO MAKE THE WRAPS

1. Heat 1 tablespoon of sesame oil in a large skillet over medium-high heat and sauté the pork until cooked through, about 8 minutes.
2. Add the sauce and stir until it is thickened, about 4 minutes.
3. With a slotted spoon, remove the pork to a plate and set aside.
4. Wipe the skillet with a paper towel and heat the remaining 1 tablespoon of oil over medium-high heat.
5. Sauté the garlic and ginger until softened, about 3 minutes.
6. Add the bell pepper, carrot, and scallion and sauté until they are softened, about 5 minutes.
7. Return the pork to the skillet with any sauce on the plate, stirring to combine.
8. Spoon the hot pork filling into the lettuce leaves and serve.

MAKE AHEAD: Make the pork filling in advance and store sealed in the refrigerator for up to 4 days. The filling is also delicious cold, so spoon it directly into lettuce leaves and serve.

PER SERVING: Calories: 383; Total Fat: 31g; Total Carbohydrates: 6g; Net Carbs: 4g; Fiber: 2g; Protein: 20g; Erythritol Carbs: 3g
MACROS: Fat: 73% / Carbs: 6% / Protein: 21%

Slow Cooker Buffalo Pork with Blue Cheese Dressing

SERVES 4 / PREP TIME: 10 MINUTES / COOK TIME: 6 HOURS ON LOW

5-INGREDIENT, 500 CALORIES OR FEWER, NUT-FREE

The classic combination of hot buffalo sauce and blue cheese is applied to pork chops in this set-it-and-forget-it preparation. Your taste buds won't be disappointed.

2 tablespoons extra-virgin olive oil, divided

1 pound pork center loin chop, cut into 1½-inch chunks

1 cup hot sauce

¼ cup melted butter

¼ cup water

1 teaspoon minced garlic

½ cup Blue Cheese Dressing (page 160)

1. Grease the insert of a slow cooker with 1 tablespoon of olive oil.
2. Place a large skillet over medium-high heat and add the remaining 1 tablespoon of olive oil.
3. Brown the pork, about 5 minutes, and transfer it to the slow cooker insert.
4. In a small bowl, whisk together the hot sauce, butter, water, and garlic.
5. Pour the mixture over the pork. Cover the slow cooker with its lid and cook on low for 6 hours.
6. Serve topped with the Blue Cheese Dressing.

VARIATION TIP: If you don't have a slow cooker, you can also make this recipe in the oven. Simply brown the pork and place it in a casserole dish, pour the sauce over, and bake, covered, until very tender, about 1½ hours at 350°F.

PER SERVING: Calories: 402; Total Fat: 33g; Total Carbohydrates: 3g; Net Carbs: 3g; Fiber: 0g; Protein: 22g
MACROS: Fat: 75% / Carbs: 3% / Protein: 22%

Sesame Pork Spareribs

**SERVES 4 / PREP TIME: 10 MINUTES, PLUS 30 MINUTES MARINATING TIME /
COOK TIME: 3½ TO 4 HOURS**

ALLERGEN-FREE

Pork and sesame oil go together like blue jeans and a white shirt. Sesame oil, known as the queen of oils, contains potent antioxidants that have benefits both inside and outside the body. This recipe also works with pork chops (instead of ribs) if you reduce the cook time to 30 minutes in a 400°F oven.

½ cup low-sodium chicken broth

3 tablespoons sesame oil

3 tablespoons apple cider vinegar

2 tablespoons coconut aminos

2 tablespoons granulated erythritol

1 teaspoon minced garlic

1 teaspoon peeled grated fresh ginger

2 pounds pork spareribs, membranes peeled off

2 tablespoons roasted sesame seeds, for garnish

1. Preheat the oven to 250°F.
2. In a large bowl, stir together the chicken broth, sesame oil, apple cider vinegar, coconut aminos, erythritol, garlic, and ginger and add the ribs to the bowl, turning to coat.
3. Marinate the ribs for 30 minutes; then transfer the ribs to a baking sheet with a lip and cover with aluminum foil.
4. Bake the ribs until very tender, 3½ to 4 hours, to an internal temperature between 190°F and 200°F.
5. While the ribs are baking, pour the marinade into a small saucepan and bring to a boil over medium heat. Reduce the heat to low and simmer until the sauce is syrupy and thick, about 5 minutes.
6. Baste the ribs every 30 minutes with the sauce, cover them back up, and continue baking until done.
7. Serve topped with the sesame seeds.

MAKE AHEAD: After cooking, portion the ribs, pour the marinade into freezer-safe bags, and seal. Freeze for up to 3 months and cook from frozen in a 400°F oven until fully warm, 35 to 40 minutes.

PER SERVING: Calories: 672; Total Fat: 60g; Total Carbohydrates: 2g; Net Carbs: 1g; Fiber: 1g; Protein: 32g; Erythritol carbs: 6g
MACROS: Fat: 80% / Carbs: 1% / Protein: 19%

Italian Sausage Ratatouille

SERVES 4 / PREP TIME: 15 MINUTES / COOK TIME: 45 MINUTES

1 PAN/1 POT, 500 CALORIES OR FEWER, ALLERGEN-FREE

Ratatouille is a French stew originating in Provence, a region known for bountiful vegetables. The stew is usually vegetarian, but spiced Italian sausage enhances the typical eggplant, peppers, zucchini, tomatoes, and garlic comprising this dish. Plus adding that meat helps dial in your keto macros.

3 tablespoons extra-virgin olive oil

1 pound Italian sausage meat

½ eggplant, cut into ½-inch cubes

2 zucchini, diced

1 red bell pepper, diced

½ red onion, chopped

1 tablespoon minced garlic

1 (15-ounce) can low-sodium diced tomatoes

1 tablespoon chopped fresh basil

1 tablespoon balsamic vinegar

Pinch red pepper flakes

Sea salt

Freshly ground black pepper

2 teaspoons chopped fresh oregano, for garnish

1. Heat the olive oil in a large stockpot over medium-high heat and sauté the sausage until it is cooked through, about 7 minutes.
2. Add the eggplant, zucchini, bell pepper, onion, and garlic and sauté until the vegetables are softened, about 10 minutes.
3. Stir in the tomatoes, basil, balsamic vinegar, and red pepper flakes and bring the mixture to a boil.
4. Reduce the heat to low and simmer until the vegetables are tender, about 25 minutes.
5. Season with salt and pepper and serve topped with the oregano.

SUBSTITUTION TIP: For a vegetarian dish, omit the Italian sausage and top the cooked ratatouille with mozzarella or crumbled goat cheese. You can also add a fried egg atop the finished vegetable stew.

PER SERVING: Calories: 429; Total Fat: 33g; Total Carbohydrates: 12g; Net Carbs: 8g; Fiber: 4g; Protein: 21g
MACROS: Fat: 70% / Carbs: 10% / Protein: 20%

Beef Bacon Burgers

SERVES 8 / PREP TIME: 10 MINUTES / COOK TIME: 15 MINUTES

30-MINUTE, 500 CALORIES OR FEWER

These are bacon cheeseburgers—yes—but with cheese inside the meat, not melted on top. There's just something fun about biting into a pocket of Cheddar. Freeze these patties raw or cooked and store for up to 3 months. Try freezing them on a baking sheet so that you won't have to chisel away at a solid hunk of beef.

1 pound grass-fed ground beef

8 ounces bacon, chopped

¼ cup ground pecans

¼ cup chopped onion

1 large egg

2 ounces Cheddar cheese, diced

¼ teaspoon sea salt

Pinch freshly ground black pepper

1 tablespoon extra-virgin olive oil

Favorite keto-friendly burger toppings

1. Preheat a grill to medium-high. (Or preheat an oven to 450°F.)
2. In a medium bowl, combine the beef, bacon, pecans, onion, egg, Cheddar cheese, salt, and pepper until well mixed.
3. Form the beef mixture into 8 equal patties and brush them with the olive oil.
4. Grill the burgers, turning once until cooked through, 13 to 15 minutes in total. (If using an oven, place the patties on a baking sheet lined with parchment paper and bake until cooked through, turning once, about 20 minutes in total.)
5. Serve with your favorite toppings.

VARIATION TIP: Use ground chicken, pork, turkey, lamb, or bison instead of beef. Keep everything else the same.

PER SERVING: Calories: 315; Total Fat: 27g; Total Carbohydrates: 1g; Net Carbs: 0g; Fiber: 1g; Protein: 18g
MACROS: Fat: 75% / Carbs: 2% / Protein: 23%

Rib Eye Steak with Anchovy Compound Butter

SERVES 4 / PREP TIME: 15 MINUTES, PLUS CHILLING TIME / COOK TIME: 10 MINUTES

1 PAN/1 POT, 5-INGREDIENT, 30-MINUTE, 500 CALORIES OR FEWER, NUT-FREE

With its distinctive marbling, rib eye is one of the fattiest cuts of beef, making it ideal for your keto diet. And rib eye with butter? This is a high-fat dish indeed! Feel free to substitute a leaner cut of steak; your macros will be fine.

¼ cup unsalted butter, at room temperature

4 anchovies packed in oil, drained and minced

1 teaspoon minced garlic

½ teaspoon freshly squeezed lemon juice

4 (4-ounce) rib eye steaks

Sea salt

Freshly ground black pepper

1. In a small bowl, stir together the butter, anchovies, garlic, and lemon juice until well blended. Chill the butter in the refrigerator until you are ready to use it.
2. Let the steaks come to room temperature.
3. Season the steaks with salt and pepper.
4. Preheat the grill to medium-high heat.
5. Grill the steak until the desired doneness, 5 minutes per side for medium-rare.
6. Let the steaks rest for 10 minutes and serve topped with the anchovy butter.

MAKE AHEAD: Make the butter ahead and freeze in a mold or rolled log for up to 3 months.

PER SERVING: Calories: 446; Total Fat: 38g; Total Carbohydrates: 0g; Net Carbs: 0g; Fiber: 0g; Protein: 26g
MACROS: Fat: 76% / Carbs: 0% / Protein: 24%

Sirloin Steak with Creamy Mustard Sauce

SERVES 4 / PREP TIME: 10 MINUTES / COOK TIME: 15 MINUTES

1 PAN/1 POT, 5-INGREDIENT, 30-MINUTE, NUT-FREE

Who has the time to cook restaurant-quality meals every night? Well, with this recipe, you do. The creamy mustard sauce makes this dish—no exaggeration—Michelin star–worthy. Just make sure you use a robust mustard in your sauce (none of that yellow mass-produced stuff).

4 (4-ounce) sirloin steaks

2 tablespoons extra-virgin olive oil

Sea salt

Freshly ground black pepper

1 cup heavy (whipping) cream

¼ cup grainy mustard

1 teaspoon chopped fresh thyme

1. Let the steaks come to room temperature.
2. Preheat the oven to broil.
3. Rub the steaks all over with the olive oil, and then season them with salt and pepper.
4. Place the steaks on a baking sheet and broil them for 7 minutes per side for medium-rare.
5. While the steaks are broiling, place a small saucepan over medium heat and pour in the heavy cream and mustard.
6. Bring the sauce to a boil; then reduce the heat to low and simmer until the sauce is very thick, 5 to 6 minutes.
7. Remove from the heat and stir in the thyme.
8. Let the steaks rest for 10 minutes before serving them topped with the mustard sauce.

SUBSTITUTION TIP: Double the sauce and save the extra in a sealed container in the refrigerator for up to 5 days. Reheat it in a skillet and pour over fish, poultry, pork, or roasted vegetables for a real treat.

PER SERVING: Calories: 505; Total Fat: 43g; Total Carbohydrates: 2g; Net Carbs: 2g; Fiber: 0g; Protein: 24g
MACROS: Fat: 78% / Carbs: 1% / Protein: 21%

Traditional Fried Steak and Eggs

SERVES 2 / PREP TIME: 5 MINUTES / COOK TIME: 20 MINUTES

1 PAN/1 POT, 5-INGREDIENT, 30-MINUTE, DAIRY-FREE, NUT-FREE

Packed with fat and protein and on the table in less than 30 minutes. Sounds ideal for a busy day, no? Add tomato slices, sweet melon, or berries to the plate for pizzazz and color; the extra carbs shouldn't derail your macros.

2 (4-ounce) strip loin steaks

Sea salt

Freshly ground black pepper

3 tablespoons extra-virgin olive oil, divided

4 large eggs

1 teaspoon chopped fresh parsley, for garnish

1. Bring the steaks to room temperature and season them all over with salt and pepper.
2. Heat 2 tablespoons of olive oil in a large skillet over medium-high heat.
3. Panfry the steaks, 6 to 7 minutes per side for medium-rare.
4. Remove the steaks from the skillet and set aside to rest for 10 minutes.
5. Heat the remaining 1 tablespoon of oil in the skillet on medium-low heat and crack in the eggs.
6. Fry the eggs until the whites are set but the yolks are still runny, about 4 minutes.
7. Serve 1 steak and 2 eggs per person, garnished with the parsley.

ADDITION TIP: Add sautéed cooked sweet potato and onion to this dish to round out the breakfast theme. A half cup of diced sweet potato, a quarter cup of chopped onion, and 1 tablespoon of olive oil per portion adds 183 calories, changing the macros to Fat: 72% / Carbs: 8% / Protein: 20%.

PER SERVING: Calories: 547; Total Fat: 44g; Total Carbohydrates: 1g; Net Carbs: 1g; Fiber: 0g; Protein: 35g
MACROS: Fat: 73% / Carbs: 0% / Protein: 27%

Grilled Flank Steak with Bacon Onion Jam

**SERVES 4 / PREP TIME: 10 MINUTES, PLUS 20 MINUTES MARINATING TIME /
COOK TIME: 10 MINUTES**

5-INGREDIENT, 30-MINUTE, ALLERGEN-FREE

Flank steak is a lean cut of beef. You need to add fat to hit your keto macros. To this end, this recipe uses a simple vinaigrette marinade, heavy on the olive oil. You can also broil the steak in the oven if you do not have a grill. Broil until desired doneness, about 7 minutes per side for medium-rare, and let rest 10 minutes.

2 tablespoons extra-virgin
  olive oil
2 tablespoons
  balsamic vinegar
1 (1-pound) flank steak
1 cup Bacon Red Onion Jam
  (page 166)
Sea salt
Freshly ground black pepper
1 teaspoon chopped
  fresh parsley

1. In a medium bowl, stir together the olive oil and balsamic vinegar and add the steak, turning to coat. Let stand at room temperature for 20 minutes.
2. Let the Bacon Red Onion Jam come to room temperature.
3. Preheat the grill to medium-high heat.
4. Remove the steak from the marinade and season the steak with salt and pepper. Discard the marinade.
5. Grill the steak until your desired doneness, about 5 minutes per side for medium-rare.
6. Remove the steak from the grill and let rest for 10 minutes before slicing the meat across the grain.
7. Serve with the Bacon Red Onion Jam.

ADDITION TIP: Add a portion of Cauliflower Pumpkin Seed Couscous (page 87) as a side dish. This creates a 1,104-calorie meal rich in fiber, protein, and fat. The new macros are Fat: 73% / Carbs: 5% / Protein: 22%.

PER SERVING: Calories: 598; Total Fat: 50g; Total Carbohydrates: 2g; Net Carbs: 2g; Fiber: 0g; Protein: 35g
MACROS: Fat: 75% / Carbs: 2% / Protein: 23%

Chile Garlic Sauce Short Ribs

SERVES 4 / PREP TIME: 10 MINUTES / COOK TIME: 2 HOURS, 10 MINUTES

1 PAN/1 POT, 5-INGREDIENT, ALLERGEN-FREE

Short ribs seem intimidating to make, but this recipe makes it easy. As an added bonus, this meat is super keto-friendly. This meal can also be prepared on the stovetop in a covered skillet; just simmer the ribs for 2½ hours or until they are fall-off-the-bone tender.

4 (4-ounce) beef short ribs
Sea salt
Freshly ground black pepper
1 tablespoon extra-virgin olive oil
2 cups low-sodium beef broth
1 cup Chile Garlic Sauce (page 161)

1. Preheat the oven to 325°F.
2. Lightly season the beef ribs with salt and pepper.
3. Heat the olive oil in a deep oven-safe skillet with a lid over medium-high heat.
4. Pan sear the ribs on all sides until browned, about 10 minutes in total, and stir in the beef broth and Chile Garlic Sauce. Bring the liquid to a boil.
5. Cover the skillet and braise the ribs in the oven until the meat is fall-off-the-bone tender, about 2 hours. Serve.

ADDITION TIP: If you're eating one meal a day, swap the Chile Garlic Sauce for a buttery Buffalo hot sauce in the same amount. This takes the calories to over 900 per serving. Serve the ribs with a salad topped with Everyday Balsamic Dressing (page 158) and enjoy!

PER SERVING: Calories: 718; Total Fat: 66g; Total Carbohydrates: 1g; Net Carbs: 1g; Fiber: 0g; Protein: 30g
MACROS: Fat: 80% / Carbs: 0% / Protein: 20%

"Pasta" Carbonara

SERVES 6 / PREP TIME: 10 MINUTES / COOK TIME: 15 MINUTES

30-MINUTE, 500 CALORIES OR FEWER, NUT-FREE

Carbonara was created in Italy during World War II. Powdered eggs and bacon (the two main ingredients) were staple wartime rations. After the war, returning GIs brought carbonara back to the United States, and it soon caught on in restaurants and kitchens everywhere. Carbonara sauce might not be in your usual keto repertoire, but it's quick and delicious, so you should make the leap.

8 bacon slices, chopped
1 tablespoon minced garlic
½ cup dry white wine
4 large egg yolks
2 large eggs
½ cup heavy (whipping) cream
2 tablespoons chopped fresh parsley
2 tablespoons chopped fresh basil
½ cup grated Parmesan cheese, divided
Sea salt
Freshly ground black pepper
4 medium zucchini, spiralized

1. Cook the bacon in a large skillet over medium-high heat, about 6 minutes.
2. Add the garlic and sauté for 3 minutes.
3. Stir in the white wine to deglaze the skillet, about 2 minutes. While the bacon is cooking, whisk the egg yolks, eggs, heavy cream, parsley, basil, and ¼ cup of Parmesan cheese in a small bowl until well mixed.
4. Season the egg mixture with salt and pepper and set aside.
5. Add the zucchini noodles to the skillet with the bacon, reduce the heat to low, and sauté for 2 minutes.
6. Add the egg mixture to the skillet and toss until well combined and the egg sauce is cooked through and thick, about 4 minutes.
7. Serve topped with the remaining ¼ cup of Parmesan cheese.

ADDITION TIP: Double the portion size to create a meal that's 658 calories. The fat and protein in the recipe keep you satiated, but because the base is light zucchini, you won't feel overly full.

PER SERVING: Calories: 329; Total Fat: 26g; Total Carbohydrates: 7g; Net Carbs: 5g; Fiber: 2g; Protein: 19g
MACROS: Fat: 71% / Carbs: 6% / Protein: 23%

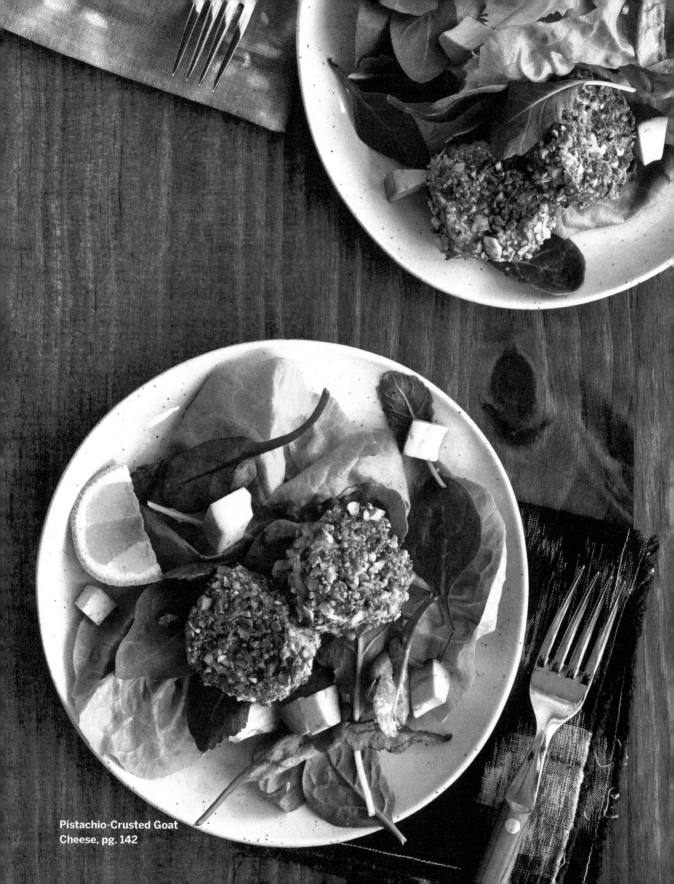

Pistachio-Crusted Goat
Cheese, pg. 142

CHAPTER NINE

Small Meals & Fast-Friendly Beverages

Smoked Salmon Deviled Eggs

SERVES 5 / PREP TIME: 20 MINUTES

5-INGREDIENT, 30-MINUTE, 500 CALORIES OR FEWER, DAIRY-FREE, NUT-FREE

Deviled eggs were a staple party food in the '70s, but the origins of this dish stretch all the way back to ancient Rome. Back then, Romans served hardboiled eggs in a creamy sauce as an appetizer. The term "deviled eggs" came later and simply refers to the spices adorning this snack. Deviled eggs are the perfect addition to a salad and can be useful on fasting days when you need to limit calories.

5 large hardboiled eggs
¼ cup Simple Mayonnaise (page 165) or store-bought
3 ounces smoked salmon, chopped
½ teaspoon Dijon mustard
¼ teaspoon chopped fresh dill
Freshly ground black pepper

1. Halve each of the eggs lengthwise and carefully remove the yolks.
2. Place the yolks in a medium bowl and place the whites, hollow-side up, on a plate.
3. Mash the yolks with a fork and stir in the mayonnaise, smoked salmon, mustard, and dill until very well mixed.
4. Season the mixture with pepper.
5. Spoon the mixture into the egg white halves.
6. Store the eggs, covered, in the refrigerator for up to 1 day.

VARIATION TIP: For a vegetarian version, omit the smoked salmon and add avocado, curry powder, sun-dried tomato, or hot peppers. Feel free to experiment.

PER SERVING: Calories: 179; Total Fat: 15g; Total Carbohydrates: 1g; Net Carbs: 1g; Fiber: 0g; Protein: 10g
MACROS: Fat: 75% / Carbs: 3% / Protein: 22%

Jalapeño Lunch Poppers

SERVES 4 / PREP TIME: 20 MINUTES / COOK TIME: 15 MINUTES

NUT-FREE, VEGETARIAN

Most roadhouse restaurant menus have some sort of deep-fried jalapeño popper, but these poppers are much healthier. And yes, the cheese cools down the hot peppers nicely. Depending on your fasting plan, you'll only need a couple to meet your caloric needs. To increase the protein, stir in a scoop of unflavored protein powder with the cheeses. You won't even notice it's there.

4 large jalapeño peppers

4 ounces cream cheese, at room temperature

4 ounces goat cheese, at room temperature

1 scallion, green parts only, finely chopped

2 tablespoons chopped fresh cilantro

¼ teaspoon garlic powder

⅛ teaspoon red pepper flakes

½ cup shredded Cheddar cheese

1 tablespoon chopped fresh parsley, for garnish

1. Preheat the oven to 400°F.
2. Line a baking sheet with parchment paper and set aside.
3. Cut the jalapeño peppers in half lengthwise and scoop out the seeds and insides of each and discard. Set the jalapeños on the prepared baking sheet.
4. In a medium bowl, stir together the cream cheese, goat cheese, scallion, cilantro, garlic powder, and red pepper flakes until well combined.
5. Evenly divide the filling among the pepper halves and top each with the Cheddar cheese.
6. Bake until the peppers are softened, the filling is bubbly, and the cheese topping is golden brown, 12 to 14 minutes.
7. Serve topped with the parsley.

MAKE AHEAD: Make the filling 3 to 4 days in advance and spoon it into the peppers just before you serve them. The filling is also delicious in mushroom caps, cherry tomatoes, and endive spears.

PER SERVING: Calories: 245; Total Fat: 21g; Total Carbohydrates: 3g; Net Carbs: 2g; Fiber: 1g; Protein: 11g
MACROS: Fat: 77% / Carbs: 5% / Protein: 18%

Pistachio-Crusted Goat Cheese

SERVES 4 / PREP TIME: 20 MINUTES / COOK TIME: 5 MINUTES

5-INGREDIENT, 30-MINUTE, 500 CALORIES OR FEWER, VEGETARIAN

Goat cheese is a soft cheese with a chalky texture that holds its shape when heated. If you're using hard or semi-hard goat cheeses, be aware that these products do contain carbs, so take the time to check the nutrition label.

¼ cup almond flour

1 large egg, beaten with 2 tablespoons water

3 ounces finely chopped pistachios

1 teaspoon chopped fresh thyme

1 (4-ounce) log goat cheese

1 tablespoon extra-virgin olive oil

1. Place the almond flour on a plate and place the bowl with the beaten egg next to the almond flour. Combine the pistachios and thyme on another plate next to the egg.
2. Cut the goat cheese using a thin thread or wire into 8 equal rounds.
3. Dredge a goat cheese round in the almond flour, then the egg, and then the pistachios, covering the goat cheese completely.
4. Set the coated goat cheese aside and repeat with the remaining rounds.
5. Heat the olive oil in a large skillet over medium heat and panfry the goat cheese rounds, turning carefully once, until lightly browned on both sides, about 5 minutes in total.
6. Serve immediately.

ADDITION TIP: Add a simple salad topped with oil and vinegar to these golden beauties for a 500-calorie meal. You'll love how nice the plate looks.

PER SERVING: Calories: 279; Total Fat: 23g; Total Carbohydrates: 6g; Net Carbs: 4g; Fiber: 2g; Protein: 12g
MACROS: Fat: 74% / Carbs: 8% / Protein: 18%

Cheese-Crusted Portobello Mushrooms

SERVES 4 / PREP TIME: 10 MINUTES / COOK TIME: 20 MINUTES

30-MINUTE, VEGETARIAN, 500 CALORIES OR FEWER

These golden baked mushrooms are an ideal small meal, but they also make a lovely starter. Alternatively, use smaller baby portobellos to create hors d'oeuvres for guests and family. To bulk up the dish, add sautéed spinach or kale to the mushroom hollow before topping with cheese and nuts.

¼ cup extra-virgin olive oil

2 tablespoons balsamic vinegar

Sea salt

Freshly ground black pepper

4 medium portobello mushrooms, stemmed and the black gills scooped out

¼ cup ground almonds

¼ cup shredded Asiago cheese

1 tablespoon freshly chopped basil

1 tablespoon freshly chopped oregano

4 ounces shredded mozzarella cheese

1. Preheat the oven to 400°F. Line a baking sheet with parchment paper and set aside.
2. In a medium bowl, stir together the olive oil and balsamic vinegar and season lightly with salt and pepper.
3. Add the mushrooms to the dressing and toss to coat.
4. Place the mushrooms on the baking sheet hollow-side up and roast until tender, about 12 minutes.
5. While the mushrooms are roasting, stir together the ground almonds, Asiago cheese, basil, and oregano in a small bowl.
6. Remove the mushrooms from the oven and carefully tip out and discard any liquid collecting in the hollows. Evenly divide the mozzarella cheese among the hollows and top with the almond mixture.
7. Bake the mushrooms until the cheese and topping are golden and bubbly, about 5 minutes.

ADDITION TIP: Serve these cheesy mushrooms with a portion of Spaghetti Squash Egg Bake (page 97) for a 635-calorie meal. The earthy mushrooms combine well with the sweet flavor of squash.

PER SERVING: Calories: 282; Total Fat: 22g; Total Carbohydrates: 8g; Net Carbs: 5g; Fiber: 3g; Protein: 13g
MACROS: Fat: 70% / Carbs: 12% / Protein: 18%

Pumpkin Pecan Fat Bombs

MAKES 12 FAT BOMBS / PREP TIME: 10 MINUTES, PLUS 30 MINUTES CHILLING TIME

30-MINUTE, 500 CALORIES OR FEWER, VEGETARIAN

These tasty nuggets are like tiny pumpkin cheesecakes: warmly spiced and slightly nutty. The combination of tart goat cheese, rich pumpkin, and buttery pecans is addictive, so double the batch to store some in the freezer for later. Swap sweet potato for pumpkin (or almonds for pecans) without significantly changing the macros.

½ cup butter, at room temperature

½ cup goat cheese, at room temperature

1 teaspoon granulated erythritol

¼ teaspoon ground cinnamon

¼ teaspoon ground nutmeg

½ cup pure pumpkin purée

¼ cup finely chopped pecans

1. In a medium bowl, stir together the butter, goat cheese, erythritol, cinnamon, and nutmeg until very smooth.
2. Stir in the pumpkin purée and pecans until well blended.
3. Place the mixture in the refrigerator until it is firm enough to roll into balls, about 30 minutes.
4. Use a tablespoon to measure the fat bombs and roll them into balls. Place the balls in the freezer in an 8-by-8-inch baking dish until very firm.
5. Transfer them to a container with a lid and store in the freezer for up to 1 month.

MAKE AHEAD: Enjoy these fat bombs right from the freezer. Two of these delicious morsels will net you 200 calories and 20 grams of fat.

PER SERVING (1 FAT BOMB): Calories: 100; Total Fat: 10g; Total Carbohydrates: 1g; Net Carbs: 0g; Fiber: 1g; Protein: 1g; Erythritol Carbs: 0g

MACROS: Fat: 90% / Carbs: 6% / Protein: 4%

Buttery Bacon Fat Bombs

MAKES 12 FAT BOMBS / PREP TIME: 20 MINUTES, PLUS 30 MINUTES CHILLING TIME

30-MINUTE, 500 CALORIES OR FEWER, NUT-FREE

When a craving strikes, what could be better than two types of cheese, hot peppers, and crispy bacon? Make sure you blot the oil off the bacon bits with a paper towel before rolling the balls to help your fat bombs stick to the baking dish. Don't worry. This step doesn't affect the macros.

4 ounces goat cheese, at room temperature

2 ounces shredded sharp Cheddar cheese

¼ cup butter, at room temperature

1 teaspoon finely chopped scallion, green part only

Pinch red pepper flakes

8 bacon slices, cooked and finely chopped

1. Line a 9-by-9-inch baking dish with parchment paper and set aside.
2. In a medium bowl, stir together the goat cheese, Cheddar cheese, butter, scallion, and red pepper flakes until well combined.
3. Place the mixture in the refrigerator until it is firm enough to roll into balls, about 30 minutes.
4. Place the chopped bacon in a small bowl.
5. Use a tablespoon to measure the fat bombs and roll them into balls. Roll the balls in the chopped bacon, covering them.
6. Place the fat bombs in the baking dish and place in the freezer until the fat bombs are very firm.
7. Store the fat bombs in a sealed container for up to 1 month.

CRAVING TIP: Bacon and cheese satisfy salty and savory cravings, guaranteed. The 13 grams of fat and 8 grams of protein also fill you up right.

PER SERVING (1 FAT BOMB): Calories: 149; Total Fat: 13g; Total Carbohydrates: 0g; Net Carbs: 0g; Fiber: 0g; Protein: 8g
MACROS: Fat: 79% / Carbs: 1% / Protein: 20%

Chipotle Chocolate Fat Bombs

**MAKES 12 FAT BOMBS / PREP TIME: 10 MINUTES, PLUS 1 HOUR CHILLING TIME /
COOK TIME: 5 MINUTES**

5-INGREDIENT, 30-MINUTE, 500 CALORIES OR FEWER, NUT-FREE, VEGETARIAN

Centuries ago, the Mayans and Aztecs believed chocolate and chile to be foods fit for gods. They consumed the two ingredients without sweetener but with a little vanilla to mellow the bitterness. This fat bomb is even better. Increase the erythritol if you prefer a dessert-like creation, but remember that a little erythritol goes a long way.

¾ cup coconut oil

¼ cup butter, at room temperature

¼ cup cocoa powder

2 teaspoons granulated erythritol

⅛ teaspoon chipotle chili powder

1. Place a medium saucepan over low heat and combine the coconut oil, butter, cocoa powder, erythritol, and chili powder in the pan.
2. Heat, whisking, until the ingredients are melted and well mixed, about 3 minutes.
3. Pour the mixture evenly into 12 mini metal or silicone muffin cups.
4. Place the muffin cups into the refrigerator until very firm, about 1 hour.
5. Pop the fat bombs out of the muffin cups and transfer them to a container. Store in the freezer for up to 1 month.

VARIATION TIP: If you don't like chile, omit the chili powder and add ¼ teaspoon cinnamon and ¼ teaspoon vanilla. For another variation, add ½ teaspoon espresso powder.

PER SERVING: Calories: 166; Total Fat: 18g; Total Carbohydrates: 1g; Net Carbs: 0g; Fiber: 0g; Protein: 0g; Erythritol Carbs: 0g
MACROS: Fat: 98% / Carbs: 2% / Protein: 0%

Classic Bulletproof Coffee

SERVES 1 / PREP TIME: 5 MINUTES

1 PAN/1 POT, 5-INGREDIENT, 30-MINUTE, 500 CALORIES OR FEWER, NUT-FREE, VEGETARIAN

Non-keto folks may recoil at the idea of adding straight fat to their precious coffee, but they've never tried this creation. It's thick, creamy, and similar to a latte without the added sugar. Use grass-fed butter for an extra nutrient-dense boost of creaminess. This beverage will fill you up, keep you full, and power your day with clean, stable energy.

1½ cups hot brewed coffee
2 tablespoons grass-fed unsalted butter
1 tablespoon MCT oil
¼ teaspoon vanilla extract

Combine the coffee, butter, MCT oil, and vanilla in a blender and blend until smooth and creamy. Serve immediately.

SUBSTITUTION OR VARIATION TIP: Add a teaspoon of cocoa powder to make a mocha beverage, or substitute a teaspoon of hazelnut extract for the vanilla to make an exciting coffeehouse creation. Enjoy breaking your fast.

PER SERVING: Calories: 333; Total Fat: 37g; Total Carbohydrates: 0g; Net Carbs: 0g; Fiber: 0g; Protein: 0g
MACROS: Fat: 100% / Carbs: 0% / Protein: 0%

Spiced Bulletproof Coffee

SERVES 1 / PREP TIME: 5 MINUTES

1 PAN/1 POT, 30-MINUTE, 500 CALORIES OR FEWER, NUT-FREE, VEGETARIAN

Most coffeehouse beverages are packed with sugar and additives—definitely not recommended for keto fasting. Never fear because the coffee, healthy fats, spices, and coconut milk in this brew will scratch your coffeehouse itch. Sit back, inhale the warm spices, and enjoy your blend.

1 cup hot brewed coffee
¼ cup coconut milk
2 tablespoons grass-fed unsalted butter
1 tablespoon MCT oil
1 tablespoon granulated erythritol (optional)
¼ teaspoon ground cinnamon
Pinch ground ginger
Pinch ground nutmeg

Combine the coffee, coconut milk, butter, MCT oil, erythritol (if using), cinnamon, ginger, and nutmeg in a blender and blend until smooth and creamy. Serve immediately.

CRAVING TIP: Cinnamon, researchers have found, can help stabilize blood sugar. This is good news for lowering sugar cravings and stabilizing appetite.

PER SERVING: Calories: 483; Total Fat: 51g; Total Carbohydrates: 4g; Net Carbs: 2g; Fiber: 2g; Protein: 2g
MACROS: Fat: 95% / Carbs: 3% / Protein: 2%

Keto Tea (Latte)

SERVES 1 / PREP TIME: 5 MINUTES

1 PAN/1 POT, 5-INGREDIENT, 30-MINUTE, 500 CALORIES OR FEWER, VEGETARIAN

Bulletproof Coffee is good stuff. Why not substitute tea for coffee? It has the same richness from the butter and MCT oil—just like a latte. Omit the almond milk if you want a more undiluted tea flavor.

1½ cups hot
  strong-brewed tea
½ cup unsweetened
  almond milk
2 tablespoons grass-fed
  unsalted butter
1 tablespoon MCT oil
1 tablespoon granulated
  erythritol (optional)

Combine the tea, almond milk, butter, MCT oil, and erythritol (if using) in a blender and blend until smooth and creamy. Serve immediately.

VARIATION TIP: Try different teas in this latte and see which becomes a favorite! You can also use different nut milks (coconut, cashew, soy) and spices such as cinnamon, ginger, nutmeg, and cayenne to add depth and complexity to the brew. Here are some suggestions: chai / matcha / green tea / Earl Grey / rooibos / peppermint / Darjeeling / oolong / chamomile / rosehip.

PER SERVING: Calories: 359; Total Fat: 39g; Total Carbohydrates: 1g; Net Carbs: 0g; Fiber: 1g; Protein: 1g
MACROS: Fat: 98% / Carbs: 1% / Protein: 1%

Vegan Bulletproof Coffee Latte

SERVES 1 / PREP TIME: 5 MINUTES

1 PAN/1 POT, 5-INGREDIENT, 30-MINUTE, 500 CALORIES OR FEWER, DAIRY-FREE, VEGAN

Bulletproof Coffee was invented by Dave Asprey, the founder of Bulletproof. Feel free, however, to use non-Bulletproof ingredients. Vegan Bulletproof Coffee Latte is less thick than the original (no butter!) but still contains MCT oil, or medium-chain triglycerides. This easily metabolized fat is thought to help burn fat, promote mental clarity, and curb sugar cravings.

1½ cups hot brewed coffee
½ cup unsweetened almond milk
2 tablespoons MCT oil
¼ teaspoon vanilla extract

Combine the coffee, almond milk, MCT oil, and vanilla in a blender and blend until smooth and creamy. Serve immediately.

ADDITION TIP: Go ahead and top this rich beverage with a whopping spoonful of whipped coconut cream. Welcome to coffeehouse heaven. The cream also adds fat and calories, about 10 grams of fat and 100 calories per ¼ cup.

PER SERVING: Calories: 278; Total Fat: 30g; Total Carbohydrates: 1g; Net Carbs: 0g; Fiber: 1g; Protein: 1g
MACROS: Fat: 96% / Carbs: 2% / Protein: 2%

Bulletproof Chili Cocoa

SERVES 1 / PREP TIME: 10 MINUTES / COOK TIME: 5 MINUTES

30-MINUTE, VEGETARIAN

When you need some serious energy for your day, blend up a mug of this cocoa and hit the floor running. This tastes like a dessert but has tons of health benefits thanks to the cacao. If you prefer a less sweet variation, reduce the erythritol to a teaspoon or so.

¾ cup unsweetened almond milk

¼ cup coconut milk

3 tablespoons cocoa powder

2 tablespoons grass-fed unsalted butter

1 tablespoon granulated erythritol

1 tablespoon MCT oil

¼ teaspoon vanilla extract

Pinch chili powder

1. In a small saucepan, bring the almond milk and coconut milk to a boil over high heat, about 4 minutes.
2. Pour the hot liquid into a blender and add the cocoa powder, butter, erythritol, MCT oil, vanilla, and chili powder and blend until creamy and smooth.
3. Serve immediately.

ADDITION TIP: If you're doing OMAD, combine this beverage with Layered Egg Bake (page 53), Pork Pumpkin Ragout (page 124), or Chicken Tenders with Creamy Almond Sauce (page 118) to get 1,000 to 1,200 calories per day.

PER SERVING: Calories: 571; Total Fat: 55g; Total Carbohydrates: 14g; Net Carbs: 7g; Fiber: 7g; Protein: 5g; Erythritol Carbs: 12g
MACROS: Fat: 87% / Carbs: 9% / Protein: 4%

Mint Strawberry Soda

SERVES 2 / PREP TIME: 10 MINUTES

5-INGREDIENT, 30-MINUTE, 500 CALORIES OR FEWER, ALLERGEN-FREE, VEGAN

Sometimes you need a fizzy treat to get through the day. Unfortunately, store-bought sodas either are packed with sugar or contain artificial sweeteners. Skip them and make this berry-infused beverage instead. Strawberries are very high in several essential nutrients such as ellagic acid, beta-carotene, potassium, and vitamins A, B, C, and E. Vitamin E is an important antioxidant that benefits skin health.

1 cup halved strawberries
¼ cup fresh mint leaves
¼ cup freshly squeezed lemon juice
1 to 2 tablespoons granulated erythritol
3 cups sparkling water
Ice cubes
Mint sprigs, for garnish

1. Combine the strawberries, mint, lemon juice, and erythritol in a blender and blend until smooth.
2. Pour the strawberry mixture through a fine sieve into a pitcher and pour in the sparkling water, stirring to combine.
3. Serve immediately over ice and garnished with the mint sprigs.

CRAVING TIP: This beverage isn't strictly keto, but it still has only 4 net carbs per serving. Keep a pitcher in the refrigerator for up to 3 days to curb cravings without derailing your diet.

PER SERVING: Calories: 37; Total Fat: 1g; Total Carbohydrates: 6g; Net Carbs: 4g; Fiber: 2g; Protein: 1g; Erythritol Carbs: 6g
MACROS: Fat: 24% / Carbs: 64% / Protein: 12%

Coconut Lime Milkshake

SERVES 2 / PREP TIME: 5 MINUTES

1 PAN/1 POT, 30-MINUTE, 500 CALORIES OR FEWER, DAIRY-FREE, VEGETARIAN

This beverage doesn't contain milk, but it's just as creamy as a real milkshake, so the name seemed appropriate. Look for full-fat canned coconut milk and shake it well before using to prevent clumping.

1 cup coconut milk

1 cup unsweetened almond milk

1 cup mashed cooked cauliflower

¼ cup freshly squeezed lime juice

1 scoop vanilla protein powder

1 tablespoon erythritol

Zest of 1 lime

1 teaspoon vanilla extract

4 ice cubes

1. Combine the coconut milk, almond milk, cauliflower, lime juice, protein powder, erythritol, lime zest, and vanilla in a blender and blend until smooth.
2. Add the ice and blend until thick and smooth.
3. Pour into 2 glasses and serve immediately.

SUBSTITUTION OR VARIATION TIP: Swap sweet potato, pumpkin, or butternut squash for cauliflower. These sweet vegetables pair well with the coconut and citrus flavors in this drink.

PER SERVING: Calories: 337; Total Fat: 25g; Total Carbohydrates: 13g; Net Carbs: 7g; Fiber: 6g; Protein: 15g; Erythritol Carbs: 6g
MACROS: Fat: 67% / Carbs: 15% / Protein: 18%

Blueberry Yogurt Drink

SERVES 2 / PREP TIME: 5 MINUTES

1 PAN/1 POT, 30-MINUTE, 500 CALORIES OR FEWER, VEGETARIAN

Ever had kefir? This beverage tastes similar. Let's review the ingredients now. Greek yogurt is high in protein yet has only about half the sugar of regular yogurt. Blueberries (plentiful in this drink) burst with antioxidants and may help prevent the onset of chronic diseases. Blueberries also contain magnesium, copper, and vitamins C and K. Yum.

**1 cup nondairy milk
 (almond, cashew)**
1 cup plain Greek yogurt
½ cup blueberries
½ avocado, diced
2 tablespoons coconut oil
½ teaspoon vanilla extract
¼ teaspoon ground nutmeg

1. Combine the milk, yogurt, blueberries, avocado, coconut oil, vanilla, and nutmeg in a blender and blend until smooth.
2. Pour into 2 glasses and serve immediately.

SUBSTITUTION TIP: For a vegan version, swap out the Greek yogurt for full-fat coconut yogurt. Add a scoop of vegan vanilla protein powder to keep protein grams within keto parameters.

PER SERVING: Calories: 330; Total Fat: 22g; Total Carbohydrates: 15g; Net Carbs: 10g; Fiber: 5g; Protein: 18g
MACROS: Fat: 60% / Carbs: 17% / Protein: 23%

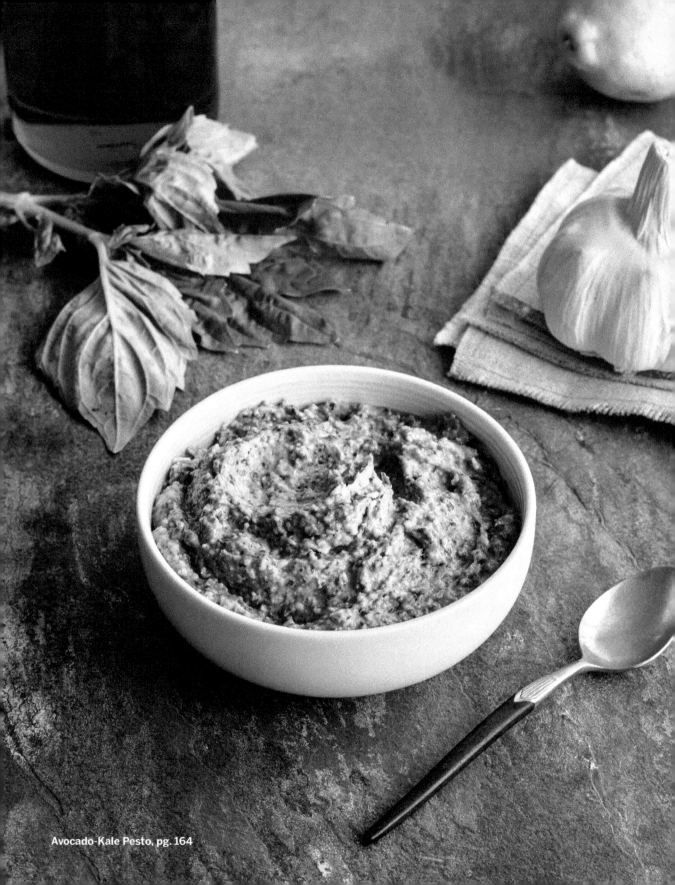

Avocado-Kale Pesto, pg. 164

CHAPTER TEN

Condiments, Sauces & Dressings

Everyday Balsamic Dressing

MAKES 1½ CUPS / PREP TIME: 5 MINUTES

1 PAN/1 POT, 5-INGREDIENT, 30-MINUTE, ALLERGEN-FREE, VEGAN

Everyone needs a go-to dressing recipe—something you can whip up when all else fails. This classic vinaigrette made with herbs, sweet balsamic vinegar, and basil fits the bill. Basil isn't just delicious; it's also a powerful antibacterial. Plus basil is a good source of vitamin K, manganese, and copper.

1 cup extra-virgin olive oil
⅓ cup balsamic vinegar
2 tablespoons chopped fresh basil
1 tablespoon chopped fresh oregano
1 teaspoon chopped fresh parsley
1 teaspoon minced garlic
Sea salt
Freshly ground black pepper

1. In a small bowl, whisk the olive oil and balsamic vinegar until emulsified, about 3 minutes.
2. Whisk in the basil, oregano, parsley, and garlic until well combined, about 30 seconds.
3. Season the dressing with salt and pepper.
4. Transfer the dressing to a container, seal, and store it in the refrigerator for up to 2 weeks.
5. Shake the dressing before using it.

VARIATION TIP: Play with the vinegar and herbs in this recipe to please your palate. Apple cider vinegar or red wine vinegar, for instance, go well with thyme, marjoram, or dill.

PER SERVING (2 TABLESPOONS): Calories: 152; Total Fat: 16g; Total Carbohydrates: 2g; Net Carbs: 2g; Fiber: 0g; Protein: 0g
MACROS: Fat: 95% / Carbs: 4% / Protein: 1%

Sesame-Ginger Dressing

MAKES 1 CUP / PREP TIME: 10 MINUTES

1 PAN / 1 POT, 5-INGREDIENT, 30-MINUTE, 500 CALORIES OR FEWER, ALLERGEN-FREE, VEGAN

Dressing? Marinade? Sauce? This fragrant creation is all three! You'll think you're in a five-star Asian restaurant when you taste the sesame oil and ginger in this dressing. Add a splash of tamari sauce to spice things up even more.

½ cup extra-virgin olive oil
¼ cup apple cider vinegar
2 tablespoons toasted sesame oil
2 tablespoons coconut aminos
1 tablespoon peeled grated fresh ginger
1 teaspoon garlic powder
1 teaspoon toasted sesame seeds

1. In a medium bowl, whisk together the olive oil, apple cider vinegar, sesame oil, coconut aminos, ginger, garlic powder, and sesame seeds until well emulsified.
2. Store the dressing in a sealed container in the refrigerator for up to 1 week.
3. Shake before using it.

MAKE AHEAD: Double or triple this recipe and store sealed in the refrigerator for a later indulgence.

PER SERVING (2 TABLESPOONS): Calories: 153; Total Fat: 16g; Total Carbohydrates: 1g; Net Carbs: 1g; Fiber: 0g; Protein: 1g
MACROS: Fat: 94% / Carbs: 3% / Protein: 3%

Blue Cheese Dressing

MAKES 2 CUPS / PREP TIME: 10 MINUTES, PLUS 2 HOURS CHILLING TIME

30-MINUTE, 500 CALORIES OR FEWER, NUT-FREE, VEGETARIAN

This is a lighter version of traditional blue cheese dressing. For a richer option, swap out the yogurt for avocado oil mayonnaise. This increases the fat but decreases protein grams.

½ cup plain Greek yogurt
½ cup sour cream
Juice of 1 lemon
1 tablespoon granulated erythritol
1 teaspoon Worcestershire sauce
½ teaspoon sea salt
½ teaspoon garlic powder
¾ cup finely crumbled blue cheese

1. In a medium bowl, stir together the yogurt, sour cream, lemon juice, erythritol, Worcestershire sauce, salt, and garlic powder until well blended.
2. Stir in the blue cheese and transfer to a container with a lid. Refrigerate for at least 2 hours before serving.
3. Store the dressing in the refrigerator for up to 1 week.

VARIATION TIP: If you enjoy smelly cheeses, use Stilton or Roquefort in this recipe. Your macros won't change much.

PER SERVING (2 TABLESPOONS): Calories: 57; Total Fat: 5g; Total Carbohydrates: 1g; Net Carbs: 1g; Fiber: 0g; Protein: 2g; Erythritol Carbs: 0g
MACROS: Fat: 78% / Carbs: 8% / Protein: 14%

Chile Garlic Sauce

MAKES 1¼ CUPS / PREP TIME: 10 MINUTES

5-INGREDIENT, 30-MINUTE, 500 CALORIES OR FEWER, ALLERGEN-FREE, VEGAN

The flavor of chiles dominates this sauce, but you'll still pick up plenty of garlic flavor. Garlic has been used for centuries as a folk remedy for immunity, digestion, and general health. Along with scores of phytochemicals, inside each garlic clove you'll find manganese, calcium, and selenium. If you're a garlic lover, double the amount in this recipe.

1 cup fresh chiles, as hot as you enjoy (jalapeño, serrano, habanero)
¼ cup apple cider vinegar
1 tablespoon extra-virgin olive oil
1 tablespoon minced garlic
1 tablespoon coconut aminos
1 tablespoon granulated erythritol
¼ teaspoon sea salt

1. Combine the chiles, apple cider vinegar, olive oil, garlic, coconut aminos, erythritol, and salt in a food processor and process until puréed.
2. Transfer to a container with a lid and store in the refrigerator for up to 2 weeks or freeze for up to 3 months.

CRAVING TIP: Did you know spicy foods can curb salt cravings? That's because spicy and salty sensations emanate from similar regions in the brain. In other words, hot sauce can kill two cravings at once.

PER SERVING (2 TABLESPOONS): Calories: 22; Total Fat: 2g; Total Carbohydrates: 1g; Net Carbs: 1g; Fiber: 0g; Protein: 0g; Erythritol Carbs: 1g
MACROS: Fat: 82% / Carbs: 16% / Protein: 2%

Enchilada Sauce

MAKES 3 CUPS / PREP TIME: 10 MINUTES / COOK TIME: 15 MINUTES

1 PAN/1 POT, 30-MINUTE, 500 CALORIES OR FEWER, ALLERGEN-FREE, VEGAN

Enchilada sauce is good for more than enchiladas. It can also be spooned over beef, chicken, pork, fish, and egg dishes. The piquant flavor works especially well with eggs, perking up their mild flavor and adding a burst of color. If you want a hotter sauce, swap the jalapeños for a hotter pepper such as habanero.

¼ cup extra-virgin olive oil
½ onion, chopped
2 jalapeño peppers, chopped
1 tablespoon minced garlic
2 cups puréed tomatoes
2 tablespoons chili powder
1 teaspoon ground cumin
1 teaspoon dried oregano
Sea salt

1. Heat the olive oil in a medium saucepan over medium-high heat.
2. Sauté the onion, jalapeños, and garlic until softened, about 4 minutes.
3. Stir in the tomatoes, chili powder, cumin, and oregano and bring the mixture to a boil.
4. Reduce the heat to low and simmer until thickened, about 10 minutes.
5. Remove the sauce from the heat and season with salt.
6. Store the sauce in a container in the refrigerator for up to 1 week.

MAKE AHEAD: Freeze for up to 1 month after chilling in the refrigerator. Store the sauce in ½-cup containers for wise portioning.

PER SERVING (¼ CUP): Calories: 65; Total Fat: 5g; Total Carbohydrates: 3g; Net Carbs: 2g; Fiber: 1g; Protein: 2g
MACROS: Fat: 70% / Carbs: 18% / Protein: 12%

Avocado-Herb Compound Butter

SERVES 12 / PREP TIME: 30 MINUTES, PLUS 4 HOURS AND 30 MINUTES CHILLING TIME

5-INGREDIENT, 30-MINUTE, NUT-FREE, VEGETARIAN

This herb-infused butter will please both your eyes and taste buds. For best results, use a ripe avocado. For faster ripening, place the avocado in a paper bag with a kiwifruit or an apple. All three fruits produce ethylene gas, a plant hormone that softens plant material.

½ cup butter, at room temperature
½ avocado, peeled, pitted and cut into quarters
Juice from ½ lime
1 tablespoon chopped fresh basil
2 teaspoons chopped fresh parsley
Sea salt
Freshly ground black pepper

1. Combine the butter, avocado, lime juice, basil, and parsley in a food processor and process until smooth.
2. Season with salt and pepper.
3. Lay a piece of plastic wrap on your work surface and spoon the butter onto the wrap.
4. Form the butter into a rough log shape and place it in the refrigerator to chill for 30 minutes.
5. Press the firmed butter into a smoother log shape about 2 inches in diameter, flattening the ends, and wrap in the plastic.
6. Place the butter in the refrigerator until it is firm, about 4 hours.
7. Slice the butter into ½-inch wide chunks and serve with beef, pork, fish, or chicken.
8. Store in the refrigerator wrapped tightly in plastic for up to 1 week.

MAKE AHEAD: Store compound butter frozen in logs, molds, or ice cube trays for later use. Use a hot knife to slice off discs and place them directly on grilled meats and poultry. There is no need to thaw. The hot meat will handle that.

PER SERVING: Calories: 80; Total Fat: 8g; Total Carbohydrates: 1g; Net Carbs: 0g; Fiber: 1g; Protein: 1g
MACROS: Fat: 90% / Carbs: 5% / Protein: 5%

Avocado-Kale Pesto

MAKES 2 CUPS / PREP TIME: 15 MINUTES

1 PAN/1 POT, 30-MINUTE, DAIRY-FREE, VEGAN

The secret to this pesto? Freshly squeezed lemon juice. This special ingredient prevents the avocado purée from oxidizing and turning a dull gray. Lemons are a good source of vitamin C along with the potent antioxidant limonene.

1 avocado, diced
1 cup chopped kale
½ cup fresh basil leaves
½ cup pine nuts
3 garlic cloves
1 tablespoon freshly squeezed lemon juice
2 teaspoons nutritional yeast
¼ cup extra-virgin olive oil
Sea salt

1. Combine the avocado, kale, basil, pine nuts, garlic, lemon juice, and nutritional yeast in a food processor and pulse until finely chopped, about 2 minutes.
2. With the food processor running, drizzle the olive oil into the pesto until a thick paste forms, scraping down the sides at least once. Season with salt.
3. Store the pesto in a sealed container in the refrigerator for up to 1 week.

MAKE AHEAD: Pesto freezes well, so whip up a batch and freeze away for future use. Pop out a pesto cube (if using ice cube trays) and drop into your soup for an instant hit of flavor.

PER SERVING (2 TABLESPOONS): Calories: 92; Total Fat: 8g; Total Carbohydrates: 3g; Net Carbs: 2g; Fiber: 1g; Protein: 2g
MACROS: Fat: 78% / Carbs: 13% / Protein: 9%

Simple Mayonnaise

MAKES 2 CUPS / PREP TIME: 10 MINUTES

1 PAN/1 POT, 5-INGREDIENT, 30-MINUTE, 500 CALORIES OR FEWER, DAIRY-FREE, NUT-FREE, VEGETARIAN

Why make your own mayonnaise when you can easily buy it? Two reasons. First, homemade tastes better. Second, you have complete control over the ingredients—no soybean oil, canola oil, peanut oil, or any other inflammatory vegetable oils. When making this mayo, use a milder olive oil or a mixture of olive oil and avocado oil to avoid a strong olive flavor.

1 large egg
2 tablespoons apple cider vinegar
1 tablespoon Dijon mustard
¾ cup extra-virgin olive oil
Sea salt
Freshly ground black pepper

1. Combine the egg, apple cider vinegar, and mustard in a blender and process until very smooth and blended.
2. Keep the blender running and slowly add the olive oil in a very thin stream until the mayonnaise is completely emulsified, about 8 minutes in total.
3. Season with salt and pepper.
4. Keep in the refrigerator in an airtight container for up to 5 days.

ADDITION TIP: Add a tablespoon or two of mayonnaise to your meals to boost fat grams and balance your macros. Mayo goes with everything!

PER SERVING (2 TABLESPOONS): Calories: 94; Total Fat: 10g; Total Carbohydrates: 0g; Net Carbs: 0g; Fiber: 0g; Protein: 1g
MACROS: Fat: 96% / Carbs: 0% / Protein: 4%

Bacon Red Onion Jam

MAKES 2 CUPS / PREP TIME: 10 MINUTES / COOK TIME: 45 MINUTES

1 PAN/1 POT, 500 CALORIES OR FEWER, ALLERGEN-FREE

This isn't technically a jam, but the natural sugars in the onion and vinegar will have you fooled. Feel free to use a sweet onion instead of a red one, but know you'll sacrifice the jam's color. Onions of all kinds are high in quercetin—a flavonoid shown to support the cardiovascular system.

2 tablespoons extra-virgin olive oil
1 red onion, chopped
2 teaspoons minced garlic
1 pound cooked bacon, chopped
½ cup low-sodium beef broth
¼ cup balsamic vinegar
¼ cup granulated erythritol
Pinch ground cloves

1. Heat the olive oil in a medium skillet over medium-high heat.
2. Sauté the onion and garlic until lightly caramelized, about 6 minutes. Reduce the heat to low and cook until the onions are completely caramelized, stirring occasionally, about 10 minutes more.
3. Increase the heat to medium and stir in the bacon, beef broth, vinegar, erythritol, and cloves.
4. Cook, stirring occasionally, until the mixture is thick and the liquid is reduced, about 30 minutes.
5. Remove the jam from the heat and let cool.
6. Store in a sealed container in the refrigerator for up to 1 week.

CRAVING TIP: Sweet, salty, savory, and slightly tart—that about sums up this sauce. Add a spoonful to wraps, proteins, soup, and stews, or stir into mayonnaise for a tempting dip. The easiest way to end cravings is to satisfy them. This jam will do just that.

PER SERVING (2 TABLESPOONS): Calories: 122; Total Fat: 10g; Total Carbohydrates: 1g; Net Carbs: 1g; Fiber: 0g; Protein: 7g; Erythritol carbs: 3g
MACROS: Fat: 74% / Carbs: 3% / Protein: 23%

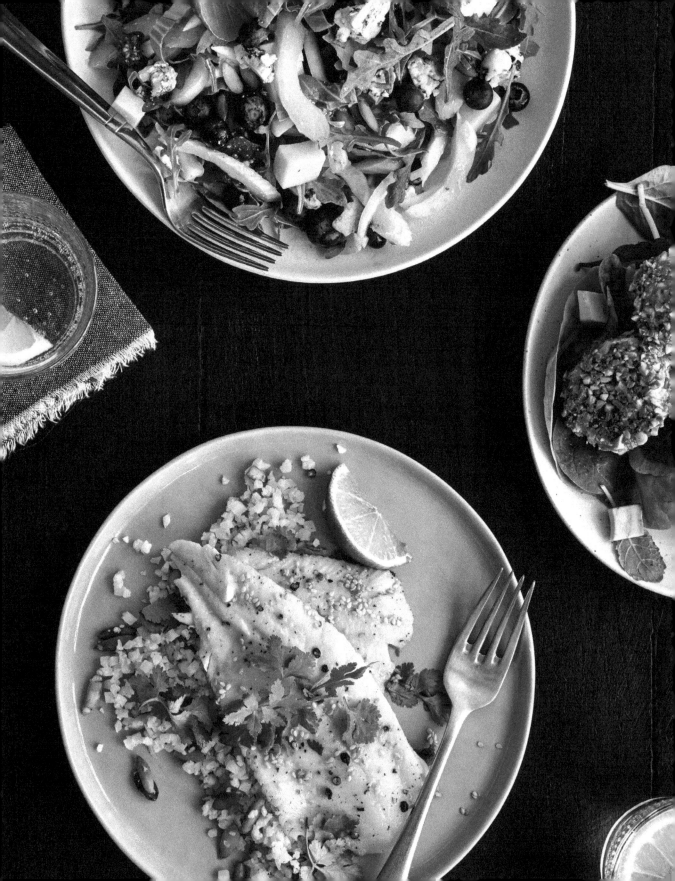

Measurement Conversions

VOLUME EQUIVALENTS (LIQUID)

US STANDARD	US STANDARD (OUNCES)	METRIC (APPROXIMATE)
2 tablespoons	1 fl. oz.	30 mL
¼ cup	2 fl. oz.	60 mL
½ cup	4 fl. oz.	120 mL
1 cup	8 fl. oz.	240 mL
1½ cups	12 fl. oz.	355 mL
2 cups or 1 pint	16 fl. oz.	475 mL
4 cups or 1 quart	32 fl. oz.	1 L
1 gallon	128 fl. oz.	4 L

OVEN TEMPERATURES

FAHRENHEIT	CELSIUS (APPROXIMATE)
250°F	120°C
300°F	150°C
325°F	165°C
350°F	180°C
375°F	190°C
400°F	200°C
425°F	220°C
450°F	230°C

VOLUME EQUIVALENTS (DRY)

US STANDARD	METRIC (APPROXIMATE)
$\frac{1}{8}$ teaspoon	0.5 mL
¼ teaspoon	1 mL
½ teaspoon	2 mL
¾ teaspoon	4 mL
1 teaspoon	5 mL
1 tablespoon	15 mL
¼ cup	59 mL
$\frac{1}{3}$ cup	79 mL
½ cup	118 mL
$\frac{2}{3}$ cup	156 mL
¾ cup	177 mL
1 cup	235 mL
2 cups or 1 pint	475 mL
3 cups	700 mL
4 cups or 1 quart	1 L

WEIGHT EQUIVALENTS

US STANDARD	METRIC (APPROXIMATE)
½ ounce	15 g
1 ounce	30 g
2 ounces	60 g
4 ounces	115 g
8 ounces	225 g
12 ounces	340 g
16 ounces or 1 pound	455 g

References

Attia, Peter. "Qualy #29—Fasting as a Powerful Drug in the Toolbox of Medicine (Sneak Peek of Paul Grewal's Upcoming Episode)." September 23, 2019. https://peterattiamd.com/qualy-29-fasting-as-a-powerful-drug-in-the -toolbox-of-medicine-sneak-peek-of-paul-grewals-upcoming-episode/.

Brehm, Bonnie J., Randy J. Seeley, Stephen R. Daniels, and David A. D'Alessio. "Randomized Trial Comparing a Very Low Carbohydrate Diet and a Calorie-Restricted Low Fat Diet on Body Weight and Cardiovascular Risk Factors in Healthy Women." *OUP Academic*. Oxford University Press. April 1, 2003. https://academic.oup.com/jcem/article/88/4/1617/2845298.

Coin, A., G. Sergi, P. Benincà, L. Lupoli, G. Cinti, L. Ferrara, G. Benedetti, G. Tomasi, et al. "Bone Mineral Density and Body Composition in Underweight and Normal Elderly Subjects." *Osteoporosis International*. U.S. National Library of Medicine. 2000. https://www.ncbi.nlm.nih.gov/pubmed/11256896.

Dhatariya, Ketan. "Blood Ketones: Measurement, Interpretation, Limitations, and Utility in the Management of Diabetic Ketoacidosis." *The Review of Diabetic Studies*. Society for Biomedical Diabetes Research. 2016. https://www.ncbi.nlm.nih.gov/pmc/articles/PMC5734222/.

Dhillon, Kiranjit K. "Biochemistry, Ketogenesis." *StatPearls [Internet]*. U.S. National Library of Medicine. April 21, 2019. https://www.ncbi.nlm.nih.gov /books/NBK493179/.

Evert, Alison B., Michelle Dennison, Christopher D. Gardner, W. Timothy Garvey, Ka Hei Karen Lau, Janice MacLeod, Joanna Mitri, et al. "Nutrition Therapy for Adults with Diabetes or Prediabetes: A Consensus Report." *Diabetes Care*. American Diabetes Association. May 1, 2019. https://care .diabetesjournals.org/content/42/5/731.

Fofaria, Neel M., Alok Ranjan, Sung-Hoon Kim, and Sanjay K Srivastava. "Mechanisms of the Anticancer Effects of Isothiocyanates." *The Enzymes*.

U.S. National Library of Medicine. 2015. https://www.ncbi.nlm.nih.gov/pubmed/26298458.

Fung, Jason, and Jimmy Moore. *The Complete Guide to Fasting: Heal Your Body through Intermittent, Alternate-Day, and Extended Fasting.* Las Vegas, NV: Victory Belt Publishing, 2016.

Grajower, Martin M., and Benjamin D. Horne. "Clinical Management of Intermittent Fasting in Patients with Diabetes Mellitus." *Nutrients.* MDPI. April 18, 2019. https://www.ncbi.nlm.nih.gov/pmc/articles/PMC6521152/.

Harvey, Cliff J. D. C., Grant M. Schofield, and Micalla Williden. "The Use of Nutritional Supplements to Induce Ketosis and Reduce Symptoms Associated with Keto-Induction: A Narrative Review." *PeerJ.* PeerJ Inc. March 16, 2018. https://www.ncbi.nlm.nih.gov/pmc/articles/PMC5858534/.

Harvie, M. N., M. Pegington, M. P. Mattson, J. Frystyk, B. Dillon, G. Evans, J. Cuzick, et al. "The Effects of Intermittent or Continuous Energy Restriction on Weight Loss and Metabolic Disease Risk Markers: A Randomized Trial in Young Overweight Women." *International Journal of Obesity* (2005). U.S. National Library of Medicine. May 2011. https://www.ncbi.nlm.nih.gov/pmc/articles/PMC3017674/.

Heilbronn, Leonie K., Steven R. Smith, Corby K. Martin, Stephen D. Anton, and Eric Ravussin. "Alternate-Day Fasting in Nonobese Subjects: Effects on Body Weight, Body Composition, and Energy Metabolism." *The American Journal of Clinical Nutrition.* U.S. National Library of Medicine. January 2005. https://www.ncbi.nlm.nih.gov/pubmed/15640462.

Ganesan, K., and Y. Habboush. "Intermittent Fasting: The Choice for a Healthier Lifestyle." *Cureus.* July 9, 2018. https://www.cureus.com/articles/12903-intermittent-fasting-the-choice-for-a-healthier-lifestyle.

Kumar, Sushil, and Gurcharan Kaur. "Intermittent Fasting Dietary Restriction Regimen Negatively Influences Reproduction in Young Rats: A Study of

Hypothalamo-Hypophysial-Gonadal Axis." *PLOS ONE*. Public Library of Science. Accessed November 20, 2019. https://journals.plos.org/plosone /article?id=10.1371/journal.pone.0052416.

Mihaylova, Maria M., Chia-Wei Cheng, Amanda Q. Cao, Surya Tripathi, Miyeko D. Mana, Khristian E. Bauer-Rowe, Monther Abu-Remaileh, et al. "Fasting Activates Fatty Acid Oxidation to Enhance Intestinal Stem Cell Function during Homeostasis and Aging." *Cell Stem Cell*. U.S. National Library of Medicine. May 3, 2018. https://www.ncbi.nlm.nih.gov/pmc /articles/PMC5940005/.

Moro, Tatiana, Grant Tinsley, Antonino Bianco, Giuseppe Marcolin, Quirico Francesco Pacelli, Giuseppe Battaglia, Antonio Palma, Paulo Gentil, et al. "Effects of Eight Weeks of Time-Restricted Feeding (16/8) on Basal Metabolism, Maximal Strength, Body Composition, Inflammation, and Cardiovascular Risk Factors in Resistance-Trained Males." *Journal of Translational Medicine*. BioMed Central. October 13, 2016. https://www.ncbi .nlm.nih.gov/pmc/articles/PMC5064803/.

Naughton, Shaan S., Michael L. Mathai, Deanne H. Hryciw, and Andrew J. McAinch. "Linoleic Acid and the Pathogenesis of Obesity." *Prostaglandins & Other Lipid Mediators*. U.S. National Library of Medicine. September 2016. https://www.ncbi.nlm.nih.gov/pubmed/27350414.

Nettleton, Jennifer A., Pamela L. Lutsey, Youfa Wang, Erin D. Michos, and David R. Jacobs. "Diet Soda Intake and Risk of Incident Metabolic Syndrome and Type 2 Diabetes in the Multi-Ethnic Study of Atherosclerosis (MESA)." *Diabetes Care*. American Diabetes Association. April 1, 2009. https://care .diabetesjournals.org/content/32/4/688.short.

Nocella, Cristina, Vittoria Cammisotto, Luca Fianchini, Alessandra D'Amico, Marta Novo, Valentina Castellani, Lucia Stefanini, Francesco Violi, and Roberto Carnevale. "Extra Virgin Olive Oil and Cardiovascular Diseases: Benefits for Human Health." *Endocrine, Metabolic & Immune Disorders Drug Targets*. U.S. National Library of Medicine. 2018. https://www.ncbi.nlm.nih .gov/pubmed/29141571.

Ota, Miho, Junko Matsuo, Ikki Ishida, Kotaro Hattori, Toshiya Teraishi, Hidekazu Tonouchi, Kinya Ashida, Takeshi Takahashi, and Hiroshi Kunugi. "Effect of a Ketogenic Meal on Cognitive Function in Elderly Adults: Potential for Cognitive Enhancement." *Psychopharmacology*. Springer Berlin Heidelberg. August 27, 2016. https://link.springer.com/article/10.1007/s00213-016-4414-7.

Paoli, Antonio, Gerardo Bosco, Enrico M. Camporesi, and Devanand Mangar. "Ketosis, Ketogenic Diet and Food Intake Control: A Complex Relationship." *Frontiers in Psychology*. Frontiers Media S.A. February 2, 2015. https://www.ncbi.nlm.nih.gov/pmc/articles/PMC4313585/.

Park, Donghwi, Jong-Hak Lee, and Seungwoo Han. "Underweight: Another Risk Factor for Cardiovascular Disease? A Cross-Sectional 2013 Behavioral Risk Factor Surveillance System (BRFSS) Study of 491,773 Individuals in the USA." *Medicine*. Wolters Kluwer Health. December 2017. https://www.ncbi.nlm.nih.gov/pmc/articles/PMC5728753/.

Patterson, Ruth E., Gail A. Laughlin, Andrea Z. LaCroix, Sheri J. Hartman, Loki Natarajan, Carolyn M. Senger, María Elena Martínez, et al. "Intermittent Fasting and Human Metabolic Health." *Journal of the Academy of Nutrition and Dietetics*. U.S. National Library of Medicine. August 2015. https://www.ncbi.nlm.nih.gov/pmc/articles/PMC4516560/.

Rains, Tia M., Sanjiv Agarwal, and Kevin C. Maki. "Antiobesity Effects of Green Tea Catechins: A Mechanistic Review." *The Journal of Nutritional Biochemistry*. U.S. National Library of Medicine. January 2011. https://www.ncbi.nlm.nih.gov/pubmed/21115335.

Regnat, K., R. L. Mach, and A. R. Mach-Aigner. "Erythritol as Sweetener—Wherefrom and Whereto?" *Applied Microbiology and Biotechnology*. Springer Berlin Heidelberg. January 2018. https://www.ncbi.nlm.nih.gov/pmc/articles/PMC5756564/.

Ruscio, Michael. *Healthy Gut, Healthy You: The Personalized Plan to Transform Your Health from the Inside Out*. Las Vegas, NV: Ruscio Institute, 2018.

Sajid, Muhammad, and Muhammad Ilyas. "PTFE-Coated Non-Stick Cookware and Toxicity Concerns: A Perspective." *Environmental Science and Pollution Research International*. U.S. National Library of Medicine, October 2017. https://www.ncbi.nlm.nih.gov/pubmed/28913736.

Sievert, Katherine, Sultana Monira Hussain, Matthew J. Page, Yuanyuan Wang, Harrison J. Hughes, Mary Malek, and Flavia M. Cicuttini. "Effect of Breakfast on Weight and Energy Intake: Systematic Review and Meta-Analysis of Randomised Controlled Trials." *BMJ* (Clinical research ed.). BMJ Publishing Group Ltd. January 30, 2019. https://www.ncbi.nlm.nih.gov/pubmed/30700403.

Simopoulos, Artemis P. "An Increase in the Omega-6/Omega-3 Fatty Acid Ratio Increases the Risk for Obesity." *Nutrients*. MDPI. March 2, 2016. https://www.ncbi.nlm.nih.gov/pmc/articles/PMC4808858/.

Solianik, Rima, Artūras Sujeta, Asta Terentjevienė, and Albertas Skurvydas. "Effect of 48 h Fasting on Autonomic Function, Brain Activity, Cognition, and Mood in Amateur Weight Lifters." *BioMed Research International*. Hindawi Publishing Corporation. 2016. https://www.ncbi.nlm.nih.gov/pmc/articles/PMC5153500/.

Solianik, Rima, and Artūras Sujeta. "Two-Day Fasting Evokes Stress, but Does Not Affect Mood, Brain Activity, Cognitive, Psychomotor, and Motor Performance in Overweight Women." *Behavioural Brain Research*. Elsevier. October 31, 2017. https://www.sciencedirect.com/science/article/pii/S0166432817314286?via=ihub.

Soliman, Ashraf, Vincenzo De Sanctis, and Rania Elalaily. "Nutrition and Pubertal Development." *Indian Journal of Endocrinology and Metabolism*. Medknow Publications & Media Pvt Ltd. November 2014. https://www.ncbi.nlm.nih.gov/pmc/articles/PMC4266867/.

Soules, M. R., M. C. Merriggiola, R. A. Steiner, D. K. Clifton, B. Toivola, and W. J. Bremner. "Short-Term Fasting in Normal Women: Absence of Effects on Gonadotrophin Secretion and the Menstrual Cycle." *Clinical Endocrinology*. U.S. National Library of Medicine. June 1994. https://www.ncbi.nlm.nih.gov/pubmed/8033362.

Stannard, Stephen R., Alex J. Buckley, Johann A. Edge, and Martin W. Thompson. "Adaptations to Skeletal Muscle with Endurance Exercise Training in the Acutely Fed versus Overnight-Fasted State." *Journal of Science and Medicine in Sport*. U.S. National Library of Medicine. July 2010. https://www.ncbi.nlm.nih.gov/pubmed/20452283.

Stote, Kim S., David J. Baer, Karen Spears, David R. Paul, G. Keith Harris, William V. Rumpler, Pilar Strycula, et al. "A Controlled Trial of Reduced Meal Frequency without Caloric Restriction in Healthy, Normal-Weight, Middle-Aged Adults." *The American Journal of Clinical Nutrition*. U.S. National Library of Medicine. April 2007. https://www.ncbi.nlm.nih.gov/pubmed/17413096.

Sumithran, P., L. A. Prendergast, E. Delbridge, K. Purcell, A. Shulkes, A. Kriketos, and J. Proietto. "Ketosis and Appetite-Mediating Nutrients and Hormones after Weight Loss." *European Journal of Clinical Nutrition*. U.S. National Library of Medicine, July 2013. https://www.ncbi.nlm.nih.gov/pubmed/23632752/.

Van Cauter, Eve, Karine Spiegel, Esra Tasali, and Rachel Leproult. "Metabolic Consequences of Sleep and Sleep Loss." *Sleep Medicine*. U.S. National Library of Medicine, September 2008. https://www.ncbi.nlm.nih.gov/pmc/articles/PMC4444051/.

Wada, Kai, Shota Yata, Osami Akimitsu, Milada Krejci, Teruki Noji, Miyo Nakade, Hitomi Takeuchi, and Tetsuo Harada. "A Tryptophan-Rich Breakfast and Exposure to Light with Low Color Temperature at Night Improve Sleep and Salivary Melatonin Level in Japanese Students." *Journal of Circadian Rhythms*. BioMed Central. May 25, 2013. https://www.ncbi.nlm.nih.gov/pmc/articles/PMC3691879/.

Wang, Bao-Hui, Qun Hou, Yu-Qiang Lu, Meng-Meng Jia, Tao Qiu, Xiao-Hang Wang, Zheng-Xiang Zhang, and Yan Jiang. "Ketogenic Diet Attenuates Neuronal Injury via Autophagy and Mitochondrial Pathways in Pentylenetetrazol-Kindled Seizures." *Brain Research*. U.S. National Library of Medicine. January 1, 2018. https://www.ncbi.nlm.nih.gov/pubmed/29056525.

Wilson, Jacob M., Ryan P. Lowery, Michael D. Roberts, Matthew H. Sharp, Jordan M. Joy, Kevin A. Shields, Jeremy Partl, Jeff S. Volek, and Dominic D'Agostino. "The Effects of Ketogenic Dieting on Body Composition, Strength, Power, and Hormonal Profiles in Resistance Training Males." *Journal of Strength and Conditioning Research*. U.S. National Library of Medicine. April 7, 2017. https://www.ncbi.nlm.nih.gov/pubmed/28399015.

Witbracht, Megan, Nancy L. Keim, Shavawn Forester, Adrianne Widaman, and Kevin Laugero. "Female Breakfast Skippers Display a Disrupted Cortisol Rhythm and Elevated Blood Pressure." *Physiology & Behavior*. U.S. National Library of Medicine. March 1, 2015. https://www.ncbi.nlm.nih.gov/pubmed/25545767.

Yang, Jai-Sing, Chi-Cheng Lu, Sheng-Chu Kuo, Yuan-Man Hsu, Shih-Chang Tsai, Shih-Yin Chen, Yng-Tay Chen, et al. "Autophagy and Its Link to Type II Diabetes Mellitus." *BioMedicine*. EDP Sciences. June 2017. https://www.ncbi.nlm.nih.gov/pmc/articles/PMC5479440/.

Resources

There are several books and websites I highly recommend for expanding your knowledge on keto, intermittent fasting, and healthy living in general.

BOOKS

The Complete Guide to Fasting by Dr. Jason Fung
Healthy Gut, Healthy You by Dr. Michael Ruscio
The Keto Reset Diet by Mark Sisson
Wired to Eat by Robb Wolf
The Paleo Cure by Chris Kresser
Keto Answers by Dr. Anthony Gustin and Chris Irvin

WEBSITES

www.chriskresser.com. Learn evidence-based health answers from functional medicine clinician Chris Kresser.

www.marksdailyapple.com. Keto advocate Mark Sisson has been covering fitness, nutrition, and everything in between on his blog here for over a decade.

www.chrismasterjohnphd.com. Take your nutrition and supplement knowledge up a notch with Dr. Chris Masterjohn.

www.peterattiamd.com. Dr. Peter Attia is on a mission to help people live healthier, more fulfilling lives. His podcast, *The Drive*, features cutting-edge commentary on fasting, keto, heart health, and much more.

www.primalsapien.com. The blog of Brian Stanton (that's me) on nutrition, longevity, meditation, and much more.

Index

Acknowledgments

You might be tempted to skip the acknowledgments section. I used to routinely skip it myself, but those days are over now. Writing my first book has made me understand: Books aren't birthed by authors alone. Some thanks are in order.

My first thank-you goes to my editor Laura Apperson for bringing me aboard, outlining the book, improving my writing, staying positive, and steering the ship from start to finish. I also need to thank Michelle Anderson for creating the recipes in this cookbook. She's a world-class recipe developer, and I was extremely fortunate to have her help.

I'm indebted as well to Mohammed Munsifzadah for finding and signing me with Callisto Media. Book deals are supposed to be painful. This was the opposite.

Finally, my biggest thanks go to my mom and dad, Peter and Christine Stanton. Their love, support, and encouragement have sustained me through life's ups and downs—and I consider myself the luckiest person on Earth to have them as parents.

About the Authors

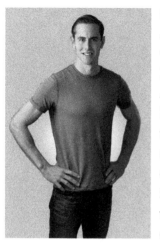

BRIAN STANTON is the author of *Keto Intermittent Fasting*, a certified health coach, and a health writer with over 150 published articles to his name. His writing has been featured in *Observer* and *Paleo Magazine*, among many other publications. Brian writes on a wide range of health-related topics including the keto diet, fasting, longevity, sleep, nutrition, fitness, and meditation—and you can find his work at www.brianjstanton.com. Brian is also the founder of www.EndingIBS.com, a website devoted to helping people overcome chronic gut issues.

MICHELLE ANDERSON is the author and ghostwriter of over 30 cookbooks focused on healthy diets and delicious food. She worked as a professional chef for over 25 years, honing her craft overseas in North Africa and all over Ontario, Canada, in fine dining restaurants. She worked as a corporate executive chef for Rational Canada for four years, collaborating with her international counterparts and consulting in kitchens all over Southern Ontario and in the United States. Michelle ran her own catering company and personal chef business and was a wedding cake designer as well. Her focus was food as medicine and using wholesome, quality field-to-fork ingredients in vibrant, visually impactful dishes. Michelle lives in Temiskaming Shores, Ontario, Canada, with her husband, two sons, two Newfoundland dogs, and three cats.